W9-BMJ-177

NO MA'AM-
OGRAMS!

Radical Rethink on Mammograms

Thank you for your interest in this work. In appreciation, Dr. Ben would like to offer you a free video series on important health issues. To receive this offer, please visit www.drbenmd.com/offer.

"There is an enormous amount of misinformation about the usefulness of mammograms. Contrary to what most physicians and public health experts will tell you, studies over the past few years have concluded that mammograms do not save lives, and may actually harm more women than they help, courtesy of false positives, overtreatment, and radiation-induced cancers. This book offers practical screening tools such as thermography and ultrasound. If you are a woman and concerned about breast cancer, this is an important read for you."

— **Dr. Mercola**, Founder Mercola.com
most visited natural health web site.

"Mammograms are lauded as a 'life-saving' tool for helping women detect breast cancer in its earliest stages. But is this the truth? Did you know that the painful compression of breast tissue during a mammogram can actually **increase** the possibility of metastasis (spreading) of cancer? Did you know that a recent Canadian study found that women who had routine mammograms before the age of 50 also had a **36% increase** in death rates from breast cancer? Are you aware that in 2009, The Cochrane Database Review found that for every **one** woman whose life is prolonged through mammography screening, that **ten** women are "unnecessarily treated" and their life is shortened? Unfortunately, we have all been sold a false bill of goods when it comes to mammograms, as the line between advertising and scientific proof has become very blurred. Truth and myths have become almost impossible to distinguish. In this groundbreaking book, *NO MA'AM-OGRAMS!*, Dr. Ben Johnson **dispels the myths** and sheds the **light of truth** on the controversial topic of mammograms, while sharing practical steps that can be taken to drastically reduce breast cancer risk. Just read it. You won't be sorry."

—**Ty Bollinger**, Author and Film Producer,
Founder of *"The Truth About Cancer"*

"It's so refreshing to see someone tell the truth about mammograms. Mammograms do not help women to keep their breasts healthy, but may actually contribute to breast disease and cancer. Dr. Ben Johnson does a wonderful job of explaining these truths. More importantly, he provides readers with many important action steps to help keep their breasts healthy and cancer-free. This book is rich with preventative tips, and highlights the importance of thermograms and ultrasounds as far safer, and more reliable alternatives to mammograms. For all women everywhere, the information in *No Ma'am-ograms!* is essential to know."

—**Christine Horner**, MD, FACS. Author of
Waking the Warrior Goddess and
Radiant Health Ageless Beauty.

"Dr. Ben Johnson's extensive expertise about integrating healing approaches is matched by his compassionate dedication to helping others regain and maintain optimal health. *No Ma'am-ograms!* is essential reading for all women and their loved ones. I highly recommend it!"

—**Larry Trivieri Jr**, bestselling author of *Alternative Medicine: The Definitive Guide*, *The Acid-Alkaline Food Guide*, and *Outstanding Health: The 6 Essential Keys To Maximize Your Energy and Well Being.*

"Dr. Johnson is right on point! Mammograms have been marketed as the gold standard – women think they are almost mandatory. In reality, routine mammogram screenings need to go the way of the dinosaur. They are late diagnostic, riddled with false readings, and are carcinogenic. We have much better methods of finding cancer long before the lump or bump. His message couldn't be more timely."

—**Jenny Hrbacek**, RN, Author of *Cancer Free! Are You SURE!*

NO MA'AM-OGRAMS!

Radical Rethink on Mammograms

by **Ben Johnson, MD, DO, NMD**

gatekeeper press

This book is intended to empower the reader with knowledge so they may begin to take responsibility for their own health. The publisher and author disclaim any liability, risk or loss, personal or otherwise, that is incurred directly or indirectly, as a consequence of the use and application of any of the contents of this book. The information herein is not intended to diagnose, treat of cure any disease. Before applying any of this book, you should seek the advice of a health care professional.

Copyright © 2016 by International Cancer Foundation Management Foundation a Panamanian S.A.

All rights reserved. In accordance with the U.S. copyright act of 1976, the scanning, uploading, and electronic sharing of any part of this book without the permission of the author constitute unlawful piracy and theft of the author's intellectual property. If you would like to use material from the book (open other than for review purposes), prior written permission must be obtained by contacting the author at info@drbenmd. com.

Thank you for your support of the author's rights.

Gatekeeper Press
3971 Hoover Rd. Suite 77
Columbus, OH 43123-2839

The publisher is not responsible for websites (or their content) that are not owned by the publisher.

Layout Design by: Mr. Merwin D. Loquias

ISBN: 9781619845381
eISBN: 9781619845398
Library of Congress Control Number: 2016949998

To Claudia Salerno, for her heroic efforts in making his project happen—from finding editors, and creating copy to doing research and infinite revisions. She's worked hours on end, above and beyond the call of duty. Thank you, Claudia; without you this project would absolutely not have come to fruition.

To Nancy Osa, my editor-in-chief. What an amazing job under pressure to complete this work! Standing ovations and cheers to you.

CONTENTS

INTRODUCTION

A Breast by Any Other Name . . .

Boobs, mammaries, bust, chest, bosom, ta-tas, "the girls," titties . . . breasts. No other appendages of the human body are so extensively nicknamed, lauded, vilified, showcased, and micromanaged. It's easy to see why the issues surrounding breast health have been so obscured. Both American women and men are fixated on breasts—not for their life-giving properties, but for a host of aesthetics whose trends have changed over time. I would like to direct your attention to matters of more importance to *you*, as an individual: the rising incidence of breast cancer, and the things you can do to welcome health and prevent disease.

You don't need to buy into the Pink Ribbon movement or mammogram marketing schemes in order to protect your well-being. Fortunately, you have the power to overcome misinformation and poor medical protocols simply by becoming more aware of your body's needs and abilities. You can learn about the growing environmental risks and take steps to avoid them. And, perhaps most importantly, you can realize that it's okay to take responsibility for the health of your breasts—in fact, you should. No one in the whole world cares more about your health and happiness than you do. This book was written solely to empower you, the owner, so read on:

The rate of breast cancer in women has increased from 1 in 22 in 1940 to 1 in 8 in 2016.

Nearly 250,000 women will be diagnosed with invasive breast cancer this year. Many of them will face debilitating radiation and chemotherapy, disfiguring biopsies and mastectomies. It's astounding that modern medicine accepts these risks as the price of restoring health. Even Hippocrates recognized this bad trade-off in 400 B.C. when he said, "It is better to give no treatment in cases of hidden cancer, as treatment causes speedy death." It seems that, with all of our medical advancements like vaccines, mammograms, CT scans, hormone therapies, birth control pills, etc., things haven't really changed that much—except for *your* risk, which has grown.

Greater exposure to radiation and carcinogenic chemicals in the environment makes the chance of getting breast cancer ever more likely. While we don't yet know of a single, definitive cause of breast cancer, we do know what many of the contributing factors are. Some of these, like your age and your family history, can't be helped. Let me state right here, though, that genetic causes of breast cancer have been dramatically overstated. Greater than 95 percent of risk factors are nongenetic and, therefore, can be controlled. All you have to do is rethink your place in the health hierarchy.

Should you trust your bodily welfare to clothing designers or insurance companies? Big Pharma or the medical establishment? The regulatory agencies of the federal government?

NO!

There are a lot of reasons *not* to place the health of your breasts in the hands of those who would profit from them. Perhaps the best one, though, is that knowing your body allows you to know what's best for it. Knowledge is power.

You can refine your diet, get more exercise, purify your water, and choose how to clothe yourself. These are key elements to your physical integrity. Just as important, you can choose to partner with a physician who understands the promotion of health, not just the eradication of disease. You can say *yes* to noninvasive monitoring systems like thermography and ultrasound, and *no* to dangerous surgical biopsies, chemical "therapies" . . . and mammograms.

Why mammograms? Simple. The U.S. Food and Drug Administration (FDA) caps radiation exposure per mammogram imaging frame at 300 millirems (mrem), so a typical four-frame test gives you 1,200 mrem, compared to 8 mrem for a single chest x-ray. That means one trip to the mammogram shop subjects you to as much as 150 times the amount of radiation as a chest x-ray. And, if you get a suspicious reading that prompts a retest, you can double that. This radiation is concentrated on a relatively small area of the body—your breasts. What's wrong with massive doses of radiation aimed directly at these important glands? Just one thing:

Radiation is one of the known causes of cancer.

If you haven't been paying attention for the past 120 years, the medical community uncovered this astounding fact during the development of x-ray imaging, when researchers were harmed or died in the course of their inquiry. Inventor Nikola Tesla suffered severe burns while studying early x-ray imaging. Madam Curie died from aplastic anemia that she developed from years of exposure to radiation. Radiographer Elizabeth Fleischman had her right arm amputated and later died from complications suffered during the evaluation of x-ray films. Wilhelm Röntgen, considered the discoverer of x-rays, died from intestinal cancer.

So, why is today's most-prescribed diagnostic test for the breasts one that employs a known risk factor for cancer? We'll talk about the driving influences behind the mammography business in Chapter 2, The Big Squeeze. What's crucial to remember is this: **you can only control your risks for breast cancer if you know what they are.** Greedy insurers and machine manufacturers, willfully ignorant doctors and lobbyists, and bureaucrats in the federal government don't want you to know. That's why you'll see "official" statistics that obscure the trends in incidence and mortality over the years. Any declines are chalked up to discontinuing dangerous hormone replacement therapy and the rise in "early detection" afforded by routine mammogram screening. We know this is a smokescreen because mammogram findings are not "early," nor are they confirmed "detection,"—only a laboratory blood test or a biopsy can definitively diagnose cancer's presence. We'll shed light on those myths in the coming chapters.

The good news is, especially in the case of breast health, knowledge is power. When you know what's wrong, you can understand what's right. When you do what's best, you take positive steps toward a long, healthy life, free of disease, with your body robust and intact.

***

But why should you focus on breast health? Well, consider that breast cancer is the main internal cancer experienced by women. Men can get it, too, but account for only about 1 percent of all diagnosed cases in the United States. This may be because female breasts are particularly vulnerable to what cancer cells "like." We know that cancer cells thrive in these body conditions:

- fatty tissue
- increased heat
- low oxygen
- acidic pH
- suppressed immune systems
- high sugar
- high toxins
- abundant estrogen
- tissue affected by radiation

Female breasts are largely made up of fatty tissue. The brassieres that most women wear insulate and confine the breasts, increasing their temperature and decreasing blood and lymph flow—substances that deliver oxygen to cells and carry toxins away. If women eat a typical diet and drink tap water, their levels of sugar, chemicals, heavy metals, and other toxic substances may be unhealthy. Add large doses of radiation to this immune-compromised body, and you've got a cancer cell's playground.

Women's risk for breast cancer, therefore, is significant—remember, one in eight, and counting. Growing environmental hazards and the forces of greed and arrogance won't be reversing that trend anytime soon. That leaves *you* as your body's most powerful advocate. You can either support breast health, or risk getting that pink slip in the mail when your body checks out.

I've spent the past twenty years of my professional career in guiding women away from misinformation and missteps, and toward self-care and empowerment. This book will give you the clarity to spot health threats and the knowledge to make informed decisions. I'll show you how to reset your thinking and stay motivated to build and maintain a healthy immune system. All you need to do is listen for the ring of truth and take the first step in the right direction.

How should you start? That's easy. Say *no, ma'am* to mammograms!

PART ONE

1 The Naked Truth

Breast Health, Breast Disease

When you look at your bustline, what do you see? Breast size, shape, and consistency vary on a wide spectrum—small to large, round to triangular, firm to floppy. Texture and appearance may change during the month, or remain consistent for years on end. The question I often hear is, *What's normal?*

This question is based on both practical curiosity and impractical fear. Girls and women want to know how their bodies compare to others'. They may see bare breasts only in brief locker-room glimpses, in fashion magazines, or in the movies and use them as standards for rating their own beauty. In the interest of better health, now is the time to abandon unrealistic comparisons to air-brushed orbs or to someone else's idea of what's attractive. The more useful question—the one that is truly meaningful—is, *What's normal for me?*

The first measure of breast health is what your breast tissue usually looks like. The second appraisal should be whether, when, and how it has changed. This is the foundation of the breast self-examination (BSE)—the basic advance warning system that every female can enlist to monitor her breast health.

Starting from a baseline of your breasts' usual features, you can recognize shifts in shape, color, texture, position, and internal qualities. These naturally occur at different life stages in most women, but they can also indicate developing problems and a need for assessment. We'll talk more about BSEs in Chapter 10.

But, let's back up for a moment. If visual and tactile clues help determine the difference between breast *health* and *disease*, you'll need to understand what those two states mean to the owner of a female body—and how the breasts, themselves, can mirror overall physical condition. In this chapter, we'll look at both sides of that health equation. We'll talk about what's normal, and what might be cause for concern. And we'll talk about the actual mechanisms behind breast illness, as well as how the hormone estrogen and estrogen-like substances can serve the body for good or evil.

***

Good to know . . .

Biopsy, surgical removal of a sample of tumor cells for diagnostic purposes.

DNA, a nucleic acid in the human body that carries genetic instructions.

Estrogen, a group of hormones (estrone, estradiol, and estriol) whose primary functions include regulating ovulation and the development of secondary sex characteristics such as breasts.

Homeostasis, a physiological balance, such as the range of blood sugar levels, needed to sustain life.

pH, a mathematical acid-base scale that measures acidity versus alkalinity: the smaller the number, the more acidic; the higher the number, the more alkaline.

Progesterone, a hormone that enables reproductive functions.

As Go the Breasts, So Goes the Body

The human body, like a book, can be broken down into distinct parts, or chapters, but it must also function as the sum of those parts. When all is well and the parts are doing their jobs, the body enjoys health, energy, and strength. The parts may work together with other features to form systems, which in turn perform important homeostatic functions, such as the regulation of pH or fluid balance. All of these intricate performances, combined, keep your body in balance and further the storyline that is your life.

Yet, bodies can tolerate some disproportion. Imbalance in one area may be compensated for by another, as when one leg becomes stronger to make up for another's shorter length or lesser muscle tone. You can even lose a limb or an organ and still survive and thrive. Harmful imbalances that occur internally or on a cellular level, though, are hard to detect. Thus, your health can slide without your knowledge—until some other clue comes to light.

In the case of breast health and illness, visible and tactile clues can definitely be good markers. Puckering of tissue, sudden disparities in size, areas of redness and heat that won't go away, and telltale lumps can all warn of possible problems. But what about what you can't see?

Dr. Bruce Lipton, a researcher and professor of cellular biology, found in a 1998 study that as much as 95 percent of all illness stems from chronic stress, which causes the immune system to malfunction. **What is stress?** Stress is a psychophysiological state that occurs when external expectations exceed internal resources to meet those expectations. In casual conversation, we use the term to mean things that make us upset or fatigued.

Those are apt metaphors for stress on the cells of your body, or groups of cells that form systems. For instance, ingesting too little salt stresses your kidneys, cardiovascular, and nervous systems. Likewise, hormone imbalances, such as too much estrogen, are known to cause stress on the immune system. It is this body system that is both integral to and an indicator of breast—and body—health.

Your immune system keeps you healthy by degrading toxins, bacteria, and viruses that enter the body, and your immune system heals you when a disease, like breast cancer, manages to take hold. Conventional medicine and surgeries can do only so much on their own. Doctors and patients must ultimately rely on the body's disease-killing mechanisms to finish the job. If your immune system is suppressed or damaged by the results of chronic stress, you will not fully recover. At the end of the day, if your immune system cannot fight off life-threatening attacks, you will not be the guest of honor at your next birthday party.

I say this not to alarm you but to show how easy it is to flip the coin between health and disease. In the case of breast health, a robust immune system is one of the keys to avoiding the conditions that promote cancer. Should you contract the disease, restoring immune system function is the right way to reinstate the body's balance that leads back to health.

The role of immunity in breast health and disease speaks to the larger issue of total body health. In other words, if you do the things that will keep your breasts in optimum condition, your overall health will benefit. That's why you'll see advice in this book related to heart, bone, and even mental health. As a bonus to keeping your breasts healthy, you may also avoid heart attacks, osteoporosis, Alzheimer's disease, diabetes, and many other sicknesses. Behind these illnesses lies mental or physical stress, which we'll explore further in Chapters 3 and 4. But first, let's define what healthy breasts are.

Perfectly Normal

Any exam starts with breast appearance; the way in which you care for your breasts, however, is related to how you view your breasts. Those two things are not the same! The first is a visual description; the second has to do with layers of social preference and pressure. These things can interfere with health maintenance.

I cannot stress enough the need to divorce yourself from images of so-called perfection that you see in the media, or that your girlfriends or boyfriends have derived from this propaganda. There is no "perfect" standard for breast beauty or vitality. In fact, those contrived standards actually promote ill health! Consider restrictive bras that use wires, latex, and plastic "bones" to push and pull breast tissue into unnatural shapes and positions. If you succumb to the pressure to "fit in" by wearing these, discomfort is the least of your worries. Researchers have actually linked certain bra-wearing habits to breast cancer, as we'll see in Chapters 3 and 7.

Additionally, trying to achieve impossible criteria dampens your self-esteem. If you view the breasts that nature gave you as lacking, your entire self-image suffers. But what do they lack? Through cosmetic, photographic, and computer tricks, the pictures of busty models or waifs with prominent nipples perpetuate *fiction.* How can you achieve what doesn't even exist? Depending on how invested you are in what others think, applying this wrong view to your own body can impair the mental processes that help you fight stress.

You'll hear more about that in later chapters. What's important to note as you set out on the road to good breast health is that **all shapes and sizes are perfectly normal.** All female breasts are composed of fatty and fibrous tissue that surrounds the milk ducts. These are served by vessels that meet inside the nipple. The outer nipple protrudes and it is encircled by an areola—skin tissue that helps stiffen the nipple to deliver milk to feeding infants. The epidermis of the areola is usually more resistant to abrasion by a sucking infant, though not in all women. The areola also has more sensory fibers allowing the release of oxytocin hormones from the brain, which causes the let-down reflex for milk production. That's what breasts were designed for.

The key factor in breast structure, then, is its purpose. I recently chatted with an acquaintance of mine who decided to stop wearing bras. Once she began to notice her breast appearance, she realized that her nipples pointed outward, and she was alarmed about this. The bras she had always worn reshaped her breasts and caused her nipples to point forward; so she thought *this* was normal. I shared with her that nipples are really supposed to point outward. Breasts were created to feed babies. It would be awkward to hold your baby out in front of you, so it's natural for nipples to point toward the crook of the arm, where a nursing baby would lie. Absolutely normal! It's fine for your lover to enjoy your breasts and for you to enjoy "owning" them. But they were created for babies, so that's why they're shaped that way.

Feel free to look at your breasts and describe them (kindly) in your own words. Are they the same size? (Most are not.) Are they flattened or rounded? Are they smooth or bumpy? Do the nipples remain erect all the time, or do they rise only when aroused? What skin colors do you see?

If you are in a state of relative health, what you see is normal, and what you see is perfect. God designed women that way. Fortunately, the physical qualities that are unique to your breasts can serve as your own personal standard of health. **Get to know what your breasts usually look and feel like,** and understand that this aspect may change:

- Over the course of your menstrual cycle
- During pregnancy
- After pregnancy

- During menopause
- As you age
- Or as you get younger!

If you see changes outside of these major life events, you'll know it's time to look more closely at the health of your breasts—and of your body.

When Cells Go Rogue

Suppose you perform a BSE or your doctor examines your breasts and an abnormality is discovered. Don't panic! Simply take the next practical step, which is to undergo a safe medical test, such as a thermogram or ultrasound. I'll tell you more about these noninvasive alternatives to overprescribed x-rays (mammograms) and biopsies in Chapters 2 and 10. At the discovery stage, though, you'll want to avoid getting an unnecessary dose of radiation or a needle biopsy that might actually encourage cancer to grow or spread.

But, now that the possibility has been raised, you'll need to know what breast cancer is, and what it isn't. Put your fears and superstition aside and look at the issue rationally. Cancer isn't a curse. Tumors aren't always cancerous, and cancer doesn't always spread. Medical science has come a long way in identifying the process by which cells become damaged and begin the rapid division that harms the body. Let's pursue that topic by looking at healthy cell structure, first.

You know that your body is made up of trillions of tiny cells—skin cells, muscle cells, nerve cells, blood cells, and other types. Each cell stands alone yet contributes to the organism as a whole. In order to live and work, each cell receives oxygen, nutrients, and substances produced by the body, such as hormones, via the bloodstream. Given this fuel, cells perform their specialized jobs.

Cell death is a normal part of life. Aging, worn-out cells must die off in order to make room for new ones. This process is called *cell senescence.* Because the life span of a cell is much shorter than that of the body as a whole, cells must replicate themselves in order to maintain the complex web of body systems that keep you alive. What a miracle! Before they die, cells can actually generate fresh copies of themselves through the process of division. The blueprints for reconstruction are contained in your cellular DNA. Directing cell construction is the "architect" of that blueprint, a creative force which determines how the building will take place. This is called *epigenetic,* and is much more significant than DNA itself. When all goes according to genetic plan, cells divide at a reasonable pace and form exact replicas of themselves, to replace dying tissue. End of process. Short and sweet.

When cellular DNA is damaged, though—by toxins, viruses, radiation, inflammation, or other means—cell division can go awry. This condition doesn't always lead to cancer. Cancer occurs when division speeds up and persists, ignoring the usual finish line.

How common is this "mistake"? Very. With trillions of cells all bent on dividing, the odds are great that some of them will be damaged. Therefore, your body experiences imperfect growth every day. Even if you lived in a "clean room," free from environmental hazards, your internal environment could still encourage cancerous cell division, and the location could be in your breasts.

If some amount of breast cancer is likely, then, why hasn't the human race been wiped out? For that, you can thank the immune system. Elements of your white blood cells are cancer eaters, which seek out the nasty things that would destroy your DNA, or which kill cells that are already rapidly dividing.

In that case, you might ask, why do people suffer and die from cancer? For one thing, because of the scale of process: remember, you have *trillions* of cells, so imagine how many hyperactive ones might need to be euthanized. But, most significantly, poor immune-system health is common in the modern world. All of our advances in farming and technology have produced some devastating health consequences.

A weak immune response can't withstand an army of rallying cancer cells. The result is that these excess cells—which don't know when to die and require increased blood flow to feed them oxygen and nutrients—drain the body of energy. Cancer cells keep reproducing and consuming, until they are literally eating both what you need to live on and the body's own stores . . . until there's nothing left.

The reason for this anatomy and physiology lesson is that the key players in breast disease—stress, cancer, and your immune system—are the focal points of this book. Toxins in our environment agitate these players. If you can crack their code by: a) reducing stress; b) (safely!) monitoring your breasts for signs of cancer; c) supporting your immune system; and d) detoxing on a regular basis, you may not only avoid developing breast cancer, you can help change the dire statistics of its incidence in the general population. What's ironic is that humans have known how to do this for a long time. It's just that the medical community, Big Pharma, and the government agencies that serve them have obscured the facts in favor of profits.

I urge you to turn away from all the hype—of which the mammogram industry is a part—and face the truth about breast health and disease. Take a look at how your lifestyle and environment affect your immune system. Breast health is not just about "the twins." It's about bringing your mind, spirit, and body into balance.

2 The Big Squeeze

Mammograms and Better Alternatives

Before we talk about the right way to achieve and maintain breast health, we must talk about the obstacles that have been placed in your way. One would hope that, after thousands of years of medical learning and practice, healthy lifestyles would be the norm today. Sadly, pursuit of power and profits causes health care providers to misdirect patients—especially women, who have historically been on the losing end of humanity's never-ending struggle for control. Mammography is just one more pile of rocks thrown in the path to good health.

We have already identified the three starring actors in the breast cancer drama—stress, cancer cells, and your immune system. Now it's time to introduce the antihero: mammograms. Think of these as the bogus elixirs sold by snake oil salesmen. They might do some good. But they probably don't live up to the glowing advertisements.

Mammography is touted as magical imagery that can ward off breast cancer. In reality, it invites the disease by throwing together the three stars: it employs **radiation** that damages cells, which jump-starts **carcinogenic cell division** and places **stress on the immune system**. And doctors everywhere want to sell you that ticket!

The pressure to get mammograms, trust mammograms, and rely on mammograms to protect your breast health is relentless. You hear it from the news, from your doctor, and from Pink Ribbon groups. Once they've been prescribed, you get "reminder" calls from the screening labs that perform them to "schedule yours today!" I have even seen mammograms advertised on billboards.

Many women resist the sales pitch for years. Some fear tissue damage and deformation caused by the plates that compress the breasts. Some fear the radiation. They listen to their "inner knower," which says: "This can't be healthy for my breasts." Others fear what they will learn from the test results. But, for most women who are tied to an insurance plan, periodic mammograms seem inevitable, and eventually, they cave in.

Next, we'll look at the upside and the downside to mammogram testing—plus the safer alternatives—so you can decide for yourself whether to make a screening appointment. If you're too young to be part of the mammogram target market of women in their mid-forties and up, don't skip this chapter. We'll also talk about how the health care business commodifies and pushes estrogen in the form of birth control pills. That's of interest to women of childbearing age, because estrogen imbalance creates a cancer-friendly environment. Even if you don't take the pill or are postmenopausal, your estrogen balance is at risk from the hormone-like action of many substances that dominate our environment. So, read on.

***

Good to Know . . .

Tests of Anatomy
Computed tomography (CT), often called a CT or CAT scan, a three-dimensional image of a body part made by a computer from a series of cross-sectional images that are formed by exposure to x-ray radiation.
Magnetic resonance imaging (MRI), a diagnostic tool that produces computerized images of internal body tissues using a powerful magnetic field and pulses of radio waves.
Mammography, a means of producing a two-dimensional black-and-white image of breast tissue using x-ray radiation.
Ultrasound, a technique that uses vibrations above the human range of hearing to create a two-dimensional image of internal body structures.

Tests of Physiology
Thermography, a process that detects and measures variations in heat emitted by the body and transforms them into visible color pictures that can be recorded photographically.

Lies, Damn Lies, and Statistics
Mammograms: so cute, so fuzzy. If they were called breast x-rays, which is what they are, would we be as inclined to accept them? Physicians are good salespeople. They make mammograms sound simple, safe . . . and mandatory. Guess what! They're not. It's just that so much money has been invested in making and selling the equipment and training people to use it that the industry needs a steady supply of customers—whether this puts patients at risk or not. But the evidence against this tactic is building.

In fact, the American Cancer Society changed its guidelines in 2015, saying that women should begin mammogram testing at 45, not 40, as previously recommended. This is because studies proved that younger breast tissue was more susceptible to the radiation risk. Who knows what they will find out tomorrow? The truth is that radiation is radiation, and it accumulates in your body with each exposure. Thermography and ultrasound are safer screening options that don't employ radiation, and they are available now. You can say *no* to mammograms, without "missing out" on breast cancer detection.

3 Reasons to Say No, Ma'am! to Mammograms

1. Each mammogram raises breast cancer risk in premenopausal women by 1 percent.
2. Radiation exposure is cumulative, so that 10 mammograms increase breast cancer risk by 10 percent.
3. Mammograms **do not decrease** the chance of death from breast cancer.

That's right. Not only do mammograms make you more likely to get breast cancer, they increase the overall death rate from the disease by 4 percent, according to Peter Gøtzsche, PhD, of the Nordic Cochrane Center of Research. His findings were published in *The Lancet*, one of the most prestigious medical journals in the world, in January of 2000.

Yes, we've known for about two decades that **women who get mammograms are 4 percent more likely to die if they get breast cancer**—and yet, your doctor still crams them down your throat! Let me explain this a little bit. First, x-ray mammograms cause breast cancer. Second, women who get mammograms are more likely to get their breast amputated from the diagnosis of ductal carcinoma *in situ* (DCIS), a form of cancer that is noninvasive and not usually life threatening. Third, they are then subjected to chemo and radiation, increasing their likelihood of other cancers, congestive heart failure, and other diseases.

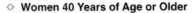

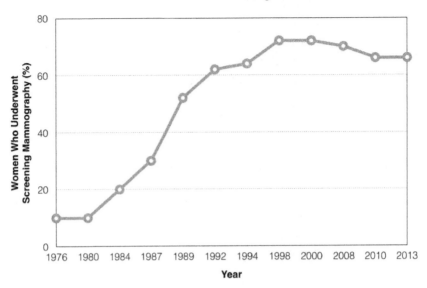

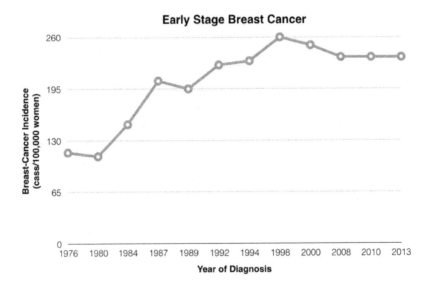

*Source: Center for Disease Control. Table 70, Health, United States, 2015 www. cdc.gov/nchs/data/hus/hus15.pdf#070 and The New England Journal of Medicine. "Effect of Three Decades of Screening Mammography on Breast-Cancer Incidence" Archie Bleyer, M.D., and H. Gilbert Welch, M.D., M.P.H. N Engl J Med 2012; 367:1998-2005. November 22, 2012.

Now let's compare what you learn about mammography from your doctor, the media, and government health sources with what is actually true. If you were to go looking for information about mammography from mainstream sources, such as the U.S. Office on Women's Health, you would find these inaccuracies promoted as "facts":
(Warning: Insert the word ***not*** after every verb!)

- Mammograms are the best method of early detection for breast cancer.
- Women between 50 and 79 years of age should have a mammogram every two years.
- Women with breast implants should have mammograms.
- The risk of harm from mammography radiation is very low.

What's wrong with those statements?

First of all, what mammograms reveal is rarely breast cancer and is not early detection. Radiologists can only see tumors in mammograms that are around 0.5 to 1 centimeter (cm) in diameter. Masses of that size contain as many as a *billion* cells. Cell number doubles during replication, which takes place about every 90 days, so—at some point—there was a first cell. This divided to make two, and those divided to make four, then sixteen, 144, and so on. In the process, some of those will have died off. So, it takes about eight to ten years for a 1 cm mass, which may or may not be cancer, to grow. That's ten years of ground gained by rogue cells before a mammogram can find out about them. *This* is considered early detection?

But, suppose the mass is cancerous. If mammograms do not find breast cancer *early*, then they could hardly be the *best* at doing so, considering there are much better tests out there. MRIs (magnetic resonance imaging) may become a good test as more doctors become better at reading them. There is a huge learning curve to a new test, and getting enough physicians adequately trained to interpret them may take years. Right now, ultrasounds and thermograms are better options than mammograms—*better* in the sense that they do no harm and provide earlier recognition of smaller groups of questionable cell masses than do mammograms. So the two parts of that "fact" are lies.

Secondly, women of any age should *not* be getting routine mammogram screening, whether annually, every two years—or at all. The ionizing radiation to which breasts are exposed is a known cause of cancer! This is a real fact, a conclusion reached again and again in peer-reviewed studies over the years. Since the mammography process typically involves four pictures, two of each breast, the amount of radiation exposure over a period of decades, added to a woman's other risk factors, can and sometimes does cause cancer.

Third, women with breast implants should *not* be getting routine mammograms, either. The efficacy of the test is reduced by the visual blockage caused by the implants. To get around this, what do radiologists do? They pry the sensitive breast tissue away from the implant and take still *more* images, each one exposing the breasts to more radiation—not to mention the possibility of rupturing the implant and causing it to leak from the compression of the plates.

Finally, to claim that the amount of radiation hurled at the breasts is insignificant is the most damaging, damning lie. When it comes to the possibility of dying, a 4-percent increase in risk is a HUGE number. **A typical four-frame mammogram generates 240 times more radiation than an airport security x-ray.** Let's say for the sake of argument that this level of radiation *might* not amount to much on its own. When you add it to a lifetime of skeletal, dental, and airport x-rays, and perhaps a CT scan or two, the amount of radiation from more than *thirty years* of mammogram screening sure as heck is significant!

So, please don't tell us that mammograms are the best, the earliest, and the safest way to detect breast cancer. The numbers don't lie.

To know how ineffective this test is, you need to know how scientists measure its results. *Sensitivity* is an assessment of how well the test finds abnormal cell masses. Is there an unusual clump of cells? *Specificity* measures how often the test correctly identifies what type of masses it finds. Are they cysts? Fibroids? Or cancerous tumors?

On a scale of 0 to 100 percent, mammograms have a 52-percent sensitivity rate in women 50 years and younger. That means they detect about half of all breast cancer masses, eight to ten years after their inception. And they do not detect inflammatory cancers—the most aggressive form—at all. Compare this track record to the sensitivity of ultrasounds, which is 74 percent, and thermograms, which is 90 percent. Both of these tests can give women far earlier warning of breast cancer development than the one test that doctors insist on, and *without* cancer-causing radiation.

And how often are mammogram readings "right"? This is a whole 'nother kettle of fish. The rate of *false negatives*—masses said not to be cancerous that later were found to be—and the rate of *false positives*—masses said to be abnormal that were not—is unacceptable. One study of specificity conducted among Harvard Medical School hospitals as of the year 2000 found that women who had received ten mammograms had a 50 percent chance of getting a false-positive result. Wrong half the time! Breast-cancer scares in half of the customers! And still the test is prescribed. Why?

That's simple, and involves another set of numbers—the kind with a dollar sign in front of them. If millions of women have annual or biannual tests for more than three decades of their lives, that's a lot of cash. Mammograms are big business, and that's why you are sold the lies.

Get It Off Your Chest

What else can go wrong as a result of mammograms' shortcomings? There are so many things; we'd better make a list.

5 More Reasons to Refuse Mammograms

1. Mammogram-plate compression can damage breast tissue or rupture cancerous tumors and cause them to spread.
2. False-positive results cause anxiety that taxes your adrenals and immune system.
3. False positives lead to needless biopsies and mastectomies.
4. False positives lead to needless radiation and chemotherapies.
5. False-negative results may cause patients to *stop* looking for cancer that is actually there!

Yes, supposedly the best test meant to prevent the scourge of breast cancer may cause affliction and death in a percentage of women who rely on it. But, what are the options? We'll talk about them in detail in Chapter 10, but here's a quick introduction.

Safe, Noninvasive Breast Screening Methods

Thermography. This test of physiology uses infrared light generated by body heat to create images of the breasts. It shows real-time activity, not just static "screenshots." So, doctors can detect changes within the breast long before a mammogram would pick them up. They can predict whether breast cancer *could* develop. This gives women a chance to take action to avoid further cancer risks and to support their immune systems in time to fight off cancer growth.
Ultrasound. This test of anatomy uses the movement of ultrasonic waves to detect cellular massing in breasts. Doctors can pair ultrasound and thermogram tests for greater sensitivity and specificity.
MRI. This anatomical test scans the breasts using magnetic fields and radio waves to find and locate solid masses. MRIs can also be paired with thermograms and ultrasounds, as necessary. MRI of the breast is a relatively new test, and not many doctors have been adequately trained in interpreting them. To give you an idea of the learning curve, physicians have been reading mammograms for over forty years, and they are just now getting real good at the technique.

Detecting conditions where breast cancer can grow or actual lumps of unidentified material is one thing; diagnosing cancer another. We'll discuss that in later chapters. The thing to remember is that **95 percent of all abnormal mammogram x-rays are NOT actually breast cancer, or are nonaggressive forms of breast cancer that will never spread.** Unfortunately, this type of "good" statistic doesn't make for snappy headlines. So, the unfounded fear surrounding breast cancer is what grows and spreads. That is the currency of the mammogram industry—fear.

In 2002, after 30 years of study, researchers in Sweden who had tracked mammography since its inception reversed their decisions about the value and harm of the test. Findings from multiple independent studies refuted numbers from within the mammography community that had been used to support screening recommendations for women beginning at age 40. The high-level Swedish task force concluded that there was no evidence of benefit for women under age 55. After a decade of widespread access to mammograms in Sweden—which should have dramatically turned the tide of cancer deaths—the mortality rate fell by only 2 percent, refuting the industry's claims that mammography was a life preserver with no measurable drawbacks.

How did mammograms become the standard? Simple. Fraud. In the initial studies done in New York and Sweden, the doctors fraudulently double counted women who didn't develop cancer and eliminated women who died from breast cancer during the trial, skewing the statistics to an amazing 31 percent decrease in breast cancer—when, in fact, the effect was the opposite. After the Nordic Cochrane Center statistically analyzed these and other studies, the numbers showed a 4 percent **increase** in death.

Mammogram screening, as a standard of a care today, is a fraud. We've known this since 1992, when a Canadian study came out showing that young women who got mammograms had a dramatic increase in the rate of breast cancer and death. Of course, these researchers were ridiculed by the people who performed the fraudulent studies. In the year 2000 when Peter Gøtzsche published in *The Lancet* showing an increased cancer rate from mammograms, he was asked, "Why would doctors do this?" Gøtzsche said, "Scientists are often driven by emotions, career aspirations, strong beliefs, money, and fame rather than facts and logic. When it comes to mammographic screening, the extent to which some scientists are ready to deny what they see and sacrifice sound scientific principles is astounding." When asked what women should do to avoid breast cancer, Gøtzsche replied, "The single most effective way to decrease women's risk of becoming a breast cancer patient is to avoid mammogram screening."

What has become crystal clear is that mammography is NOT the screening device that detects breast cancer EARLY enough to change the outcome, and worse, it has become part of the problem, increasing a woman's chance of breast cancer morbidity and mortality. This means that, to date, billions of dollars worldwide have been wasted on a breast cancer screening method that has little significance for women under age 55 and potential harm for women of any age. In 2014 the Swiss Medical Board rejected the trade-off: periodic radiation exposure plus the anxiety and harmful medical interventions prompted by false-positives for an outcome of about one cancer detection in one thousand women. They countered industry claims that the screening benefits outweighed the risks, ultimately advising that routine screening of women in Switzerland be phased out. Whether the rest of the global medical community will follow suit remains to be seen.

Estrogen, Friend or Foe?

How does the hormone estrogen affect breast tissue health? Estrogen is a blanket term for a group of hormones that kicks in during puberty to help the female body develop mature characteristics, including breast growth. It does this by encouraging tissue cells to divide and multiply more rapidly. Sound familiar?

Getting too much estrogen can "confuse" too many cells into dividing more rapidly, increasing the risk of breast cancer. One example of this state is early-onset puberty; this occurs when girls begin producing estrogen early, and so they experience greater amounts of body estrogen in their lifetimes. Another is hormone-replacement therapy (HRT), a regimen of estrogen medication which, until recently, was routinely prescribed to reduce the side effects of menopause in older women. Premarin, containing an equine hormone derived from the urine of pregnant mares, was the most famous of these medications. Climbing incidence of breast cancer among this user group revealed that HRT was a serious risk factor for breast cancer, and it has since become a last-resort therapy. Artificial hormones such as Premarin should not be confused with bioidentical HRT (BHRT), which replicate the molecular structure of human estrogens.

In a mature female body, the ovaries produce estrogen up until menopause. Other body tissues also produce smaller amounts of the hormone, which circulates through the bloodstream searching for estrogen *receptors*, or proteins on cell membranes to which it can bind. When estrogen does so in the breasts, it prompts cell division, suffering some wear and tear in the process. This "used" estrogen is released by the receptors and sent to the liver, which breaks it down for elimination from the body.

At this point, your overall health condition comes into play. If you've been eating right and avoiding environmental toxins, your liver sends the old estrogen to your colon, and it leaves your body. If your digestive health isn't all it could be, the altered estrogen is absorbed back into the bloodstream. It may wind up back in your breasts, delivering the wrong message to cells: to divide and multiply faster, and never stop.

Taking birth control pills, even on a regular schedule, interferes with this process. Hormonal balance is a tricky thing. Adding artificial estrogens or progestins (which mimic progesterone), even in low doses, may work for some women, but it may not be what *your* body needs. At the very least, birth control pills are known to cause blood clots and strokes in a percentage of women. They also contribute to depression. Some effects of this mental condition, such as insomnia and weight gain, are known to weaken the immune system. So, taking birth control pills, a known risk factor for breast cancer, can start a downward health spiral that cultivates a cancer-friendly environment.

And what happens to estrogen levels after an abortion, or at menopause? Pregnancy triggers higher estrogen production, to prepare the body for gestation, giving birth, and milk production. Abortion nips that process in the bud. And now that equine hormone-replacement therapy has been exposed as dangerous, menopausal women who have been dosing on estrogen via birth control pills for years are virtually pushed off a cliff. Their bodies, and those of women who have had abortions, are left to cope with drastically changing estrogen levels.

Then there is a problem of substances that *act* like human estrogen which bind to receptors in the breasts. These substances are called *xenoestrogens*, literally, "foreign" estrogens that are present in the environment and find their way into the human body.

What are xenoestrogens? They are hormone-like substances generated by plastics, pesticides, and other synthetic chemicals found in the world around us. They can also be hormones naturally produced by other animals. Cow-derived estrogens may be injected into livestock, whose products we then eat or drink. Equine-derived hormones may be given to women as HRTs. Unfortunately, your body can't tell the difference between xenoestrogens and the estrogens your body produces naturally. When you ingest these unnatural estrogens, they bind to your body's estrogen receptor sites and encourage unhealthy cell division.

Cells are designed to be born, fulfill their purposes, and die—not to go on living, consuming energy, and reproducing forever. Preventing the conditions in which this abnormal life cycle occurs is the best way to prevent breast cancer. I'll say it another way: **avoiding conditions that encourage rapid cell division in the breasts—and equipping your immune system to combat abnormal growth—are the best ways to prevent breast cancer.** That is a radical rethink of the prevailing medical wisdom. And that is what the rest of this book is about.

3 Home Is Where the Harm Is

Bad Stuff to Watch Out For

The environment in which you live—and how you interact with what's around you—directly affect breast health and overall well-being. Think of your surroundings in three sections, like a snail's habitat. There is the interior, vulnerable body; the outer, durable shell; and the whole, wide world beyond it. Like a snail, you have three "homes." These are:

- Your Body, or your mental, physical, and spiritual selves
- Your Home, or the house, apartment or other domicile in which you live
- Your Environment, or everything else around you

In a perfect world, these locations would all be health inducing and life sustaining. In reality, they are often the opposite! Modern life seems to throw more challenges than helping hands our way. Blame it on greed, ignorance, technology, social mores, or human weakness, as a race, we tend to derail our own survival, even though we do not wish to do so.

Instinct may tell you to seek out health advice. But it is often conflicting, limited, or just, plain wrong. So, as you set out to move away from risk and toward better breast health, make a simple and systematic plan. Divide your journey into three parts that correspond to your three "homes." Learn which dangers lurk there, and then set about avoiding, reducing, or eliminating them. You'll find a larger discussion of how to do this in the following chapters. Let's begin by identifying some of the health hazards in each home.

***

Good to know . . .

Antioxidant, a substance (such as the compound vitamin C) that prevents oxidation by harmful free-radical molecules, a process that damages cells.

Flavonoid, an antioxidant compound found in fruits, vegetables, and herbs such as grapes, onions, and parsley.

Free radical, an unstable atom/molecule that is deficient in an electron, which it steals from another atom/molecule through the process of oxidation, thereby damaging the latter atom/molecule.

Lymphatic system, part of the circulatory system that removes toxic material from the tissues of your body, returning it to the bloodstream for excretion.

Obesity, an extreme overweight condition characterized by a severely disproportionate ratio of weight to height.

Oxidation, the degrading exchange of electrons that can occur between cellular matter and free-radical atoms/molecules.

Your Body *Is* Your Temple

We all set our own boundaries for how we care for our bodies. You might not think of grooming, eating, and playing a game of tennis as activities connected to the health of your breasts, but they are. The personal care products you use, the food and water that you choose to eat, and how well you condition your muscles and bones all have long-lasting effects on the cells and systems of your body—including your breasts and your immune system. **As you make lifestyle decisions, keep the close association of breast and immune system health in mind.**

Do you smoke? Wear a padded bra? Eat a lot of meats, processed foods, or sugary/starchy foods? These are examples of choices that can harm breast health. What you take into and put on your body on a regular basis might not affect your "first home" today, but over time can add to your breast cancer risk. These hazards especially endanger women with a genetic family history of breast cancer.

It's time to clean house! Avoid, reduce, or eliminate your intake of the bad stuff. Here's a good list to start working on.

Everyday Risks to the Body, Mind, and Spirit

Cosmetics. We don't often think about it, but what we put on our skin does matter. The skin is our largest organ. It is not only an organ of excretion, getting rid of waste products through our pores when we sweat, but it also is an organ of absorption—absorbing things into the bloodstream such as water, chemicals, even drugs. The efficiency of this process is evident in a treatment for cardiac angina: topical nitroglycerin applied to the chest. It eliminates chest pain within sixty seconds!

Given the skin's amazing uptake ability, we had better be very selective about what we put on it. Read product labels, and buy all-natural makeup. We'll talk more about the toxic ingredients in cosmetics—which most have—in Chapter 9. And be careful about the type of metal that's in the jewelry that you wear right next to your skin. In 2014, fitness-minded consumers were shocked to learn that nickel in the bands of the popular Fitbit activity monitors they wore caused skin rashes. This is one symptom of metal toxicity, a known contributor to cancer. See my list of dangerous heavy metals at the end of this chapter, and wear only gold, silver, platinum, titanium, or copper pieces, which are safe for your system. Easy choice: baby your skin!

Tobacco. Smoking cigarettes causes a host of diseases, including lung cancer, by depriving your body of oxygen, in addition to the ill effects of nicotine, sugar, and other additives. Formaldehyde gas, a known cancer-causing agent, is released in tobacco smoke. Studies have shown that smoking raises your risk for breast cancer by an average of 24 percent.

The longer you smoke, the worse it gets. The American Cancer Society reports that women who started smoking before their first menstrual cycle had a 61-percent greater chance of getting breast cancer than all other women. The great news is that the moment you quit, your risk begins to decrease. Tough to do? Sure. But there are more aids than ever to help you kick the habit. Easy choice: quit!

Alcohol. Another high-risk habit is drinking alcohol. It has become *en vogue* for women to drink. Alcohol profiteers and their handlers realized they were missing half of the market share, and they went after women full force with targeted ad campaigns. Yes, red wine flavonoids are supposed to bolster heart health. But don't trade that for breast disease!

One drink a day is the cut-off point. Beyond that, you risk a 30-percent increase in the chance of developing breast cancer, according to an American Cancer Society study of nearly 250,000 women. Easy choice: limit or don't drink alcohol.

Excess weight. It might not seem right that overeating can cause malnutrition, or that both conditions contribute to breast cancer, but they do. I ask all of my cancer patients how their diets are, to which each one responds: "My diet is really pretty good." Then I ask them what their menus consist of, and I learn that they are heavy in saturated fats, trans fats, carbohydrates, and refined sugar. (This, by the way, is what the FDA considers healthy food.)

Those are things that make a person put on weight. At the same time, getting more of those nutrients usually means that you get less of the beneficial fiber, vitamins, and minerals that bolster your digestive and immune systems and actively combat cancer cells. Add couch-potato habits to the mix, and you might be headed for obesity. The American Cancer Society relates that women are more likely to develop breast cancer if they are overweight. Easy choice: pay attention to diet and exercise.

Tap Water. Do you know where your water comes from? If you're like most people, you turn on the faucet and out it comes—usually through metal or plastic pipes, from a city-drawn source that might be a nearby river or lake. The pipes themselves may taint water, as the community of Flint, Michigan, discovered in 2016, when lead leached from pipes contaminated their drinking water.

Whole bodies of water may be influenced by pesticide run-off, toxic waste from manufacturing, or even pharmaceuticals that have been flushed down the commode. Tap water is treated with chlorine and fluoride, additives that kill bacteria but do not eliminate drugs, chemicals, and pesticides that find their way into the river, lake, or aquifer. Over time, this chemical soup can wreak havoc on your immune system. You drink water every day of your life, so the source counts! Easy choice: purify your water.

Brassieres. By their very design, bras compress and heat the bust area, restricting circulation and raising body appendage temperature—two effects that make breast tissue attractive to cancer. Most women are inured to bra wearing as soon as they begin to develop breasts. Some even wear bras day and night!

Researchers have found that the longer women wear a bra during the day, the greater their risk for breast cancer. Just as significant is that some of the lowest breast cancer rates in the world are among women who live in cultures that do not include bras in everyday dress. You choose what to put on each day; you can wear a bra selectively. Easy choice: at least some of the time, ditch your bra!

Antiperspirants. Do you swab your armpits with commercial antiperspirant after putting on your bra in the morning? If so, you're sending potentially toxic metal—aluminum—directly into your lymphatic system. The lymph nodes beneath your underarms are designed to *flush* toxins from the body. Antiperspirants act to stop this mechanism.

Products that contain aluminum or that include paraben preservatives may also distort the effects of estrogen on breast tissue. Simple deodorant products, on the other hand, just cover up sweat odor. Read the labels! Easy choice: switch your sweat protection.

Negative stuff. People, places, or things that drag you down mentally or emotionally affect your physical health, too. If you have friends or relatives who are argumentative or use attacks on others' self-esteem to pump themselves up, they are sources of stress in your life. Ditto with a work or play environment that is frenetic or full of politics. (If you're a politician, you'll need special stress management!)

We'll examine in depth how the thoughts, emotions, and actions provoked by negative sources can harm your breast health in Chapter 5. It stands to reason that the opposite things—positive people or positive atmospheres—support your well-being. While we can never entirely avoid stressful situations, we can learn to cope with them and minimize their effects. Easy choice: concentrate on the positive!

Take Care of Your Backyard

The house you live in contains the air that you breathe and is the focal point for your daily routine. It's where you cook and store your food. It's where you enjoy entertainment and social interaction. You probably adorn the space, indoors and out, to reflect your personality and create pleasant surroundings in which to spend your free time. That means you make more lifestyle choices that affect your immune system and breast health.

Don't get stuck in an unhealthy rut just because you've always done things a certain way. Take the time now to ask yourself if you might improve any of your household habits. What's considered healthy, by the way, changes with the introduction of new consumer products or new information about old ones. Here's the latest scoop on a few risks to breast health that you can control.

Some Everyday Household Risks

Packaging. Watch what comes into your home when you buy products and store food and water. Xenoestrogens and other compounds that affect hormonal balance can leach from plastics and Styrofoam, particularly when these contain hot foods or liquids. We'll talk more about "good" and "bad" plastics in Chapter 6. In my opinion, though, *good* is really just *less bad*.

How often do you sip bottled water—especially water bottled in plastic—that's been left in a hot car, or a latte from a Styrofoam to-go cup? Consider healthier alternatives, like glass bottles and paper cups. Easy choice: don't heat or store food in plastic or Styrofoam.

Microwaves. Love to zap your food? You're also zapping yourself! Microwave ovens bombard food with radio waves to heat it up—as much as 2.45 billion hertz of radiation. Like other electrical appliances, they create electromagnetic fields (EMFs) that have been proven to damage human cells and body tissue.

The trouble with microwaves is that the radiation that's meant to stay in the oven leaks when door seals age, shooting out far more than we can safely absorb. That's apart from the effect it has on the cellular structure of foods. Protein is especially damaged by microwaves, making it not only unusable by the body as building material, but carcinogenic. Toaster ovens operate at a much lower frequency. Easy choice: toss the microwave.

Fertilizers, pesticides, and herbicides. Do you use Weed & Feed, Roundup, or other lawn and garden products that kill weeds and bugs? Their warning labels are extensive, and homeowners may not read them or follow their safety instructions. If you've always wondered what *Caution, Warning, and Danger* on labels really means, see the discussion of toxic ingredients in Chapter 9.

How many people make sure to apply hazardous products a safe distance from water bodies, gutters, and drainage ditches? What happens when the wrong product is sprayed or drifts onto vegetable plants, or you inhale some while applying it? The chemicals from these items work their way into the soil, water, and air around them and around you. You may literally be dosing yourself with harmful xenoestrogens. Easy choice: use lawn and garden products safely, sparingly, or not at all!

Stuff That's "Out There"

How should you handle potential threats to breast and immune system health that you *don't* control? When you leave the house and go to the doctor or to visit friends, shop downtown, or work at the office, you share the environment and all of the things in it. You're exposed to air, water, and noise pollution, unwanted radiation, and emotional pressure that can disrupt your physical and mental balance.

You may feel helpless in the face of persistent environmental and social hazards. Even when you can't control what's out there, though, you may have a choice in what space you inhabit and what you allow to contact your mind or body. If you aren't in a position to say *no*, you might be able to dictate *how much*. When you can't, you can mitigate the harm by detoxing your liver—and your mind—on a regular basis.

For now, take a look at some of the most prevalent environmental nasties you might encounter on any day. Your decisions in this realm may become more complicated to make, and their results less satisfying. But anything you can do to reduce cancer risk is a step in the right direction.

Environmental Risks

Heavy metals. We live in a metal world. From cookware to building materials to the underwire in bras, we're surrounded with the stuff. Your breast health is affected by metal molecules that are air-and water-borne, as well. Coal-fired plants and water-pipe leaching infuse the environment with toxic amounts of mercury, cadmium, arsenic, lead, nickel, and other metallic minerals. Manufacturers use certain chemicals that bond well with metal to strengthen it, sometimes increasing health risks. Cooking pans coated with Teflon and other nonstick coatings, for instance, emit fluorine gases when heated. These compounds overwhelm the body's ability to flush toxins, damaging cell structure and promoting cancerous growth.

What about metals that we choose as adornments? Because rings, necklaces, bracelets, and earrings touch the skin, bad metals and contaminants from cheap jewelry will be absorbed and poison the immune system. Do not wear accessories that have nickel or stainless steel parts. To counteract the effects of harmful metals that do find their way into your system, you should periodically cleanse the liver and colon of toxic buildup. More on that in Chapter 9. Easy choice: detox, and do not use Teflon!

X-rays and antibiotics. Doctors continue to overprescribe medical treatments that lead to breast cancer. Because the radiation that enters your body piles up over the years, you should consent to as few x-rays (including mammograms) as possible. Places where you are most likely to get unnecessary x-rays are airports, dental and chiropractic offices, and emergency rooms. Say *no* to skeletal x-rays, mammograms, and CT scans, and *yes* to safer thermograms, ultrasounds, and MRIs.

Research has also shown that cumulative antibiotic use for things like acne and chronic infections can greatly raise women's risk for breast cancer. A girl who gets six doses of antibiotics before her eighteenth birthday has a three-fold increase in breast cancer risk. Accept antibiotics only for serious bacterial infections—they don't work on the viruses that cause colds or flu! Doctors pass out antibiotics as if they were candy, both of which are bad for you. Easy choice: say *no* to unnecessary x-rays and antibiotics.

Television. How much do you watch? More importantly, what are you watching? According to Nielsen Media Research, Americans watch an average of 5 hours of TV a day. That's more than an entire day each week! The emotional stress brought on by witnessing relentless advertising and violent shows, and the physical effects of noise and sedentary behavior, compromise your immune system health. Easy choice: turn off your TV.

We'll look further at the science behind all these health threats that hit you where you live, as well as what you can do to neutralize them, in the coming chapters. Next, let's talk about the mechanism that causes so many disparate things to degrade your body and mind and increase your risk for breast cancer: stress.

4 Your Boiling Point

How Stress Contributes to Disease

You've heard about the dangers of stress and felt its effects on your mind, body, and spirit. But the whole issue still seems vague. That's because there are two major types of stress, acute and chronic, and they're used interchangeably when people talk about the subject. The collective term *stress* means different things, depending on whether it comes up in casual conversation or scientific inquiry. Let's break it down, in order to understand how stress affects your breast health.

In biological terms, stress is a cause-and-effect relationship in which an external source triggers action in the human body that prepares it to fend off an attack. The source can be a person, place, thing, or an idea that raises a red warning flag for you. The "attack"—or even just the possibility of an attack—can be verbal abuse, a tense office atmosphere, the approach of a wild animal, or worries about your bank account. Or it can even be a trigger from a past experience that you might not even recognize at the moment. Whatever poses a challenge to you can set off the stress-response mechanism in your body.

This is both a good thing and a bad thing. Humans developed this biological weapon in order to survive, back in our cavewoman days. It helped us to outsmart and outrun predators and to avoid safety problems, like getting buried in an avalanche. Today, we have fewer real survival threats of those types, and more invented ones. The media want us to worry about everything from bad breath to the zombie apocalypse, in the interest of selling us mouthwash and supplies for our underground bunkers. Manufacturers and the medical establishment assail us with hazardous plastics, metals, radiation, and all kinds of other garbage that our systems aren't designed to handle.

What does this mean to you? It means that your body's circuits for handling stress are often overloaded. What happens when the controls get jammed? Something has got to give, and your body's ability to function hangs in the balance.

***

Good to know . . .

Acute stress, a stimulus of threat or pressure that initiates the mental and physical stress response, the effects of which are fleeting.

Chronic stress, a recurrent stimulus that prompts the stress response, the effects of which are unrelenting and long term.

Stress response, a mechanism involving hormonal secretions that prepare the body to react to a threatening physical or mental challenge.

The "On" Switch

Acute stress is what first signals your body to meet a challenge. *Acute* in this sense means significant, sudden, and short-term. The trigger can be anything from a bumblebee landing on you to a bomb threat; the immediate chain of events, if not the severity of the reaction, is the same. Your heart starts pumping, your muscles tense, you breathe harder, and you begin to sweat. This is called the "fight or flight" mechanism.

How does the stress response work? When you see and hear the bee or the ticking bomb, your brain sends a hormone to the pituitary gland. The pituitary gets the message and sends another hormone to the adrenal glands. Once tagged, the adrenals release hormones you may be familiar with—including cortisol and adrenaline—into the bloodstream. Your liver dumps in some extra glucose, for energy.

At this point, you feel your body respond to the hormonal signals for your heart to beat faster, your muscles to prepare for action, and your brain to shut down lower-priority functions, such as creative thought and digestion. Switch on! You're ready to fight or take flight.

This all happens in a few seconds. Once you do what needs to be done, the cortisol in the bloodstream returns to the pituitary gland and the brain, and gives them the all-clear. If you have vanquished the threat or left it behind, they stop releasing stress hormones, and you go back to your usual physiological state.

You probably don't think about this process when you tell people that you are stressed about money, work, or relationships, but it is all happening in the background. A general feeling of stress may not be as clear-cut as your reaction to a potential bee sting or bomb scare, but the same hormones and physical effects are in play.

The Bubbling Cauldron

Let's compare that acute episode to what happens under chronic, or ongoing, stress. Suppose the threat was more than you could handle. Or maybe another problem arrived on its heels. Whatever it was, the tension did not let up, your brain and glands kept producing stress hormones, and your body kept responding to them. The physical effects that were supposed to be short-term—increased heart rate, blood pressure, blood sugar, muscle tautness, and other conditions—became the norm.

Great! You were ready for anything the cosmos might throw at you. But, as it turned out, you weren't able to resolve the problem through fighting or fleeing. Not so great. Your body wasn't meant to endure elevated levels of cortisol and adrenaline indefinitely. Those continually taut muscles might cause headaches or back pain. Sustained high blood pressure and blood sugar can put you on the road to cardiovascular disease and diabetes.

How, then, does unrelieved stress affect breast health? Circulating cortisol hormones interact with the immune system, eventually curbing normal functions. Consider college students who are stressed out during exam time for weeks on end. They tend to get flus, colds, or bronchitis. Over months or years, persistent stress can lead to depression and obesity . . . and make your body less able to fend off other diseases, like breast cancer.

Now you can see why a robust immune system is so necessary to breast health—and so elusive in today's world. With the combination of high-stress conditions plus an environment full of heavy metals and other toxins, it's a wonder people live as long as they do. That said, remember that not all stress is "bad" stress. In small doses, stress can test and improve your body's capabilities, as when you perform weight-bearing exercises that stress the bones and muscles or play Sudoku to challenge your mind. It's when you overdo things that problems arise.

Temperature Control

Relieving and managing "bad" stress, then, can support your immune system and breast health and help you prevent disease. Much of the advice in the next chapters does double duty to protect the breasts as well as to counteract chronic stress. Keeping your body and mind in good condition forms a positive loop that puts the stress response back into a context more in line with the Creator's design.

If you can relate to the destructive effects of long-term stress, you are probably overdue for some relief. Think of your body as a pressure cooker that needs to release steam before it blows. Not sure whether you're near that point? Take a look at your pressure gauge. After a long stretch of coping (or not coping) with stress, you might forget that it's even there. Aches and pains, feelings of depression, and bouts of infectious disease seem normal. The first move toward decreasing these ill effects is to recognize and acknowledge what is causing them. Make a quick mental and physical check. Do you have trouble falling asleep at night? Are your thoughts whirling, replaying conversations and situations from the day? As you lie there, try consciously relaxing your muscles, from your toes on up to your shoulders, neck, and head. Were they tight? If so, you need to dial down.

Many studies have been done about interventions that prevent stress-related disease, such as the very real benefits derived from deep breathing, laughter, and meditation. You can incorporate specific activities into your healthy routine to escape the cumulative mental and physical effects of chronic stress. Pick a favorite and stick with it, or change up your tactics—whatever it takes to make managing stress a lifelong habit. The problem is certainly not going to go away anytime soon. Here are some of my favorite ideas:

Rx for Stress

- **Walk it off.** Return to your pre-automobile ways and take a stroll. Walking when you're stressed out lets you literally move away from the source of your woes. My grandmother used to walk barefoot ten miles to school in the snow, uphill both ways. Just kidding, but you get the point.
- **Experience solitude.** You don't always need an escort or conversation partner. Many people are never alone! Spending time with yourself lets you slow down and retreat from other people's ideas, desires, needs, and pressures. It lets you recharge your personality and remember who you really are.
- **Quiet down.** Create a buffer zone in your day in which you think, look out the window, or do nothing at all. Increasing your downtime will revitalize you. Are you one of those people who can't sit still for five minutes, or who spends too much time on social networks? Turn off the TV, your phone, and the computer, and take a few moments to enjoy simply being.
- **Engage your spirit.** Pray, meditate, or connect with nature. These activities take you out of your head and away from your ego, that part of the mind that clamors for attention any way it can get some. Follow your inner knower, which will take you away from false alarms and harmful wrong beliefs—we'll talk about that in the next chapter.
- **Focus on breathing.** Spend five minutes breathing more deeply and slowly. You'll relax! Practice yoga movements or tai chi, which employ deep breathing, or pay for a session with a breath therapist. These professionals work wonders on the mind and body by facilitating the type of breathing that sends more oxygen to every cell—including those in the breasts.

- **Give and accept help.** Doing something nice for someone else is another way to take the focus off your worries and your ego's disruption. Go do something for someone who cannot do anything in return. If you're the type to suffer in silence, lighten up and let someone do something for you.

- **Reaffirm your boundaries.** Too many obligations perpetuate the stress cycle. Most perceived responsibilities are self-imposed. *You* decide how much you can handle, and say *no* to the rest.

- **Get out of the house.** Sometimes just a change of venue will knock you out of your worry rut. Connect with others, ride a bike, go fishing, or walk your dogs in the park. If you always find some excuse not to take a break, make a standing date to do so.

- **Exercise every day**. Put "good" stress to work on your "bad" stress! Research shows that any type of exercise that gets your blood pumping reduces your cortisol and adrenaline levels.

- **Grow a garden.** Studies show that growing your own garden has many benefits. It allows you to be in contact with nature, with the soil, which alone is very grounding. Planting, weeding, watering, and harvesting add purposeful physical activity. It's wonderful if you can get the kids involved to teach them about vegetables and the importance they have in our health. Your wallet, the environment, your body, and your taste buds will thank you!

- **Be conscious of your thoughts.** Your ego, like the media, thrives on contention, sending negative ideas through your stream of consciousness. During your day, notice how many times you think or say words like *hate, damn, f____, sad,* and *mad.* You can turn your frame of mind around simply by saying *love, happy, awesome, yes,* and *glad.*

PART TWO

5 Mind Matters

The Role of Thoughts and Intentions on Health

This section of the book deserves a drum roll. Now that you understand the ongoing threats to your immune system and your efforts to safeguard your breast health, it's time to focus on solutions. The chapters in Part Two all concern what you put in and on your body, and the paces that you put your body through. These pages offer specific directions on the right way to go, as you step away from risk—and toward breast health. So, get ready to take notes! You'll assess where you're at, make hard choices, and begin to form new habits. There are five major steps, involving your thoughts, diet, environment, dress, and exercise.

The first one is the Big One. You don't hear about it as often as you do pills and mammograms, because it doesn't make anybody as much money as those things do. **The first, and most important, step you can take to avoid or overcome breast cancer is to address all of emotional and spiritual issues that have become embedded in your body.** In other words, you can use mental processes to unlock what have become physical repositories for "bad stuff."

Just as your brain records things, so the cells of your body absorb information about their environment and what goes on in it. You know this simply as your life. Scientifically, it is *cellular memory*. Everything you perceive, learn, do, see, and know goes into the hopper. It all generates internal chemical reactions. The cells of your body are affected by stress hormones, inflammation, endorphins, and other substances. Your cells associate the effects of these states with past occurrences. However, your interpretations are not always correct.

Remember your ego? The attention grabber in your psyche? It does serve rational purposes of control, judgment, and memory—but, often, those powers get out of hand. Your ego urges unreasonable control, harsh judgment, and selective memory, perhaps because these tactics are less complicated than their alternatives. If you try to control everything or see things only in black and white—or don't see them at all, if you don't want to—then decisions are so much easier to make.

Unfortunately, the picture this paints for you is not real. Your mind lies. But your cells can't distinguish the difference between wishful thinking and what's true. So, among the "good stuff" in there, you are stuck with many false beliefs locked into your cellular memory. Some of these wrong convictions come from external sources—movies that you watch, people you look up to, or ideas that otherwise influence your thinking. They might also come from what someone said or didn't say, what someone did or didn't do.

What's wrong can be made right. Your mind has the power to mislead you, but it also has the power to heal you. You need only make that choice. Let's look at how tainted cellular memories become obstacles to good health, and how to surmount them.

***

Good to know . . .

Cellular memory, energy generated by cognitive memory that is stored in body cells and can be passed on epigenetically.

Epigenetics, a study of the potential for non-gene sources to affect cellular genetic expression.

Law of attraction, the theory that positive energy attracts positive energy, and negative energy attracts negative energy, which echoes the scientific perception that physical bodies in nature tend to attract or repel one another.

Your Mental Diet

You are more than a composite of all of the stimuli, events, conversations, suspicions, and criticisms that come your way. Your cells also record your *reactions* to these things, but they absorb them as facts, no matter how out of proportion they might be, once filtered through your ego. Alongside the skewed memories of your best golf game and how big your house seemed when you were a little kid sit the ugly ones. The perceived slights, failures, frights and inadequacies you've suffered are embedded in your body's cells, giving rise to anger, frustration, fear, and pain whenever some trigger dredges them up. You might consciously turn them over in your mind, and their accompanying emotions return. Or you might subconsciously retaliate for those bad feelings and lash out at someone, or even hurt yourself.

Why do you replay unpleasant events or rehash old grudges time and again? Because these things are locked in your cellular memory. Even if decades have passed and you tell yourself you don't care about those things any more, you will relive the same harmful emotions until you get rid of what causes them.

What does this have to do with breast health? Recall the link between stress, well-being, and illness. **Wrong and negative beliefs create stress, and your body responds.** You already know that the effects of prolonged stress contribute to the development of many diseases, including breast cancer. To avoid that state, then, you must eliminate the cellular memories that are at the root of your stress load.

But, that's easier said than done. You have probably been carrying that load around for a lifetime and adding to it every day. In fact, as the science of epigenetics holds, you may even have inherited some of it from your relatives.

Do you notice how much more readily your conscious memory recalls cataclysms than ordinary pleasant moments? We tend to focus on the horror, rather than the beauty, in life. Many of us, particularly women, engage in a cycle of self-destruction born of poor self-esteem. Feelings of unworthiness and other lies the mind perpetuates may come from outside ourselves, often based on the wrong beliefs of others who try to control us, rush to judgment, or deny reality. Of course, we are all guilty of doing the same thing!

So, many of your cellular memories are based on your own or other people's misinterpretations or misplaced behavior brought on by embedded anger and fear. Your mind and body absorbed those things as facts, and the negative energy that they produce adds to your stress level.

But, what else is on your mental menu? What sort of an atmosphere do you live in most of the time? What kind of input is your mind and body getting? It's time to inject some quality control into your mental and spiritual diet, because what you "eat" is truly what you are.

The Law of Attraction

If everything you see, hear, do, and are subjected to makes up your mental diet, think of your memory—cognitive and cellular—as elements of your mental digestive system. Your daily input either nourishes you . . . or drags you down. You reflect this energy through your personality and your self-image.

Thanks to thousands of years of oppression and today's social imperative to "do it all," many women struggle with self-esteem. Suppose you are one of these women. At some point in your life, an uncaring person may have told you that you were selfish, stupid, or not good enough to deserve love or respect. Comparing yourself to images in magazines and movies may have convinced you that your breasts— or your nose, or some other body part—were too small, too large, or not pretty enough.

These negative feelings spilled over and multiplied, until you repeated to yourself, "I'm such a loser! I can't do anything right. No one cares about me, and no one ever will." Clearly, these kinds of absolutes are false. No one is all bad—or all good. But you absorbed the untruths into your psyche and your body's trillions of cells, and these wrong beliefs became your physical and mental reality. Every time something else bad happened to you, it reaffirmed these lies. You came to expect the worst, and—guess what—you got it!

That is a prime example of the Law of Attraction. What you most concern yourself with is what you draw towards you. For instance, if you listen to angry talk radio shows, you end up churning with anger. If you mistrust people, others will sense it and mistrust you. If you worry continually about losing money or getting sick, those outcomes become likely. I can attest from my years of medical practice that people who are the most vocal about fearing breast cancer are the most likely to get it. They replay their fear over and over again, like a mantra, literally drawing the thing that they fear to them.

But, if negative energy attracts negative energy, the opposite must also be true.

Now, here's where the topic gets really interesting. Two different researchers came to this same conclusion through different avenues: **replacing destructive cellular memories with positive, true statements frees the body to heal disease.** Dr. Bruce Lipton performed studies at Stanford University during the 1990s that linked spiritual awakening, the power of the subconscious mind, and the body's innate healing ability. Dr. Alex Loyd, a naturopathic physician, psychologist, and Christian minister, went in search of a means for healing his wife's depression in 1996 and discovered the same thing. Both men assert that "rewiring" cellular memory relieves or eliminates chronic stress and, therefore, heals or prevents illness. I, myself, have seen proof of this theory time and again, in my medical practice and in my own life.

That's where your breast health comes in. You want to avoid the physical conditions that invite cancer cells to invade and take over your breasts and body. Why not engage your mental power to do it? I asked you back in Chapter 1 how you view your breasts—what your opinion of them is. Are you proud of them? Content with them? Or not? In other words, ask yourself what message you are sending them.

If you are at peace with your pair, that's a healthy attitude. While we're on the subject of "real ones," I urge you to accept yours as they are. Breast implants have many drawbacks—including hampering cancer diagnosis. While the term "cosmetic surgery" sounds pretty and simple, it carries the same risks as any operation performed under general anesthesia.

Breast augmentation surgery is an invasive procedure that causes stress on the body, which may get infected or reject the silicone implants and require further surgery. Of great concern is that new implants are not tested, as are other medical devices or drugs. They have been "grandfathered" under old FDA rules. So there may be significant unknown hazards due to lack of testing. Breast reduction carries similar risks. And the outcomes aren't always all roses.

Is a new profile worth the risk of scarring or nerve damage? If you're still set on augmentation, please, weigh the practical benefits and risks. But, first, consider what breast implants tell your body. Their presence suggests that something is wrong, and that's not the case. Your breasts are simply unique. If you haven't yet arrived at a state of appreciation, you may be quietly adding to your stress load.

One of the precautions you must take is to break the cycle of chronic stress and let your immune system do the job that God intended. But this requires more than lip service. You can mouth positive things as often as you like. However, until you embed them in your cellular memory **in place of the old lies**, the stress that they cause will persist in harming your body. Let's talk about how to do that.

Let the Spirit Move You

Somewhere between your mind and body lies your inner knower—the portion of you that senses the truth and importance of things and seeks to join the mental and physical in a sum that is greater than those parts. Call it your spirit, your soul, or the Divine Feminine within—it is powerful. We all sense that. It is this superior self that puts you in contact with God, or what you believe to be larger than yourself and humanity. This is what you will tap into in order to regain control over your mind and body, to banish the effects of stress and to embrace health.

It is no accident that the world's organized religions connect faith, the common good, and personal self-control. It's hard to be good, especially for the sake of God and others. Humans are wired to survive, and this usually means putting personal needs and desires first. The ability to suspend this me-first attitude requires engagement of the spirit and of the mind. When we harness these two things, we can gain mastery of our physical selves and act as we should—to move toward communion, toward the light, and toward health.

Interpreters of the ancient Chinese spiritual guide, the *I Ching*, wrote that from spiritual truth came the mental fortitude needed to make moral decisions. The power generated by this union was said to transcend the need to act or explain the good to others, because, essentially, *by one's thoughts, one commands.* This is what we are doing when we tap into cellular memory and replace false "truths" with divine ones.

How can we do this?

We must first access a cellular memory; then assess it; then consciously accept or reject it. Once we master that, we can begin to revolutionize the way in which we think, so that we are geared toward forming new, positive memories based more closely on what's true.

Let's bring this lofty concept down to Earth. The woman who believes she is not deserving of love beats herself up about it, causing herself stress and ill health. She is unable to forgive herself, based on untruths. She hurts herself. If she were to sit down in a quiet moment and think all the way back to the source of her self-loathing, she might uncover the damaging cellular memories that started the vicious cycle. Perhaps she was compared to a sibling who was perceived as more attractive, or was brutalized by a gym teacher for not being thin enough, fast enough, or strong enough. She might, in time, realize that these criteria are meaningless in her present life. She might find the grace to forgive herself for believing these lies and letting them run her life.

In the same vein, being unable or unwilling to forgive other people is a great source of stress. Many illnesses arise from the conditions caused by unforgiveness. We are not saying that forgiveness is easy—in fact, it is not! But it is necessary if we wish to lead healthy, positive lives. This is not so much because we are hurting others by not forgiving them but because we are harming ourselves. Forgiveness isn't for them; it is for ourselves. It frees us from the influence of negative people. Just how closely do you want to be connected to them anyway?

Here's an example from my life. I once loaned an acquaintance a very large sum of money. He was in a jam, and I was in a position to help him, so I gave him twenty thousand dollars with the expectation that he would pay me back. He did not. Within a week, he had filed for bankruptcy, and I realized he'd had no intention of repaying the loan. Whether he felt true remorse over this, I do not know. I, of course, was very unhappy.

In the years that followed, whenever I thought of this person, my frustration resurfaced. It was only after I'd partnered with Dr. Loyd to write *The Healing Code*, a book based on his groundbreaking work on this topic, that I realized how important it was for me to disperse these feelings, which were deeply embedded in my cellular memory. I prayed about it, utilizing my faith and Jesus's instruction to forgive our enemies, as He related in the Lord's Prayer. If we forgive others, He promised, God will forgive us.

This translates, in everyday life, to a release of negative thoughts and energy, which neutralizes stress and allows us to achieve our full potential—whether it be a just worldly existence, eternal salvation . . . or bodily health.

Realizing how important it was to my future wellness to forgive my old acquaintance, I worked on it. I made my peace with the problem, did some healing codes, and moved on. But I'm not perfect, and forgiveness is not a fixed construct. Decades have passed since that unrepaid debt in my life, yet every now and then, when that fellow pops into my mind, my first instinct it to relive the unhappiness and frustration. Clearly, I did not manage to fully exorcise the pain from my cellular memory. But that doesn't mean I've stopped trying! I simply smile, sigh, and work on forgiving him again.

I encourage you to embrace this habit. Set out to forgive those who have hurt you in the past. Sit down and make a list on paper. Recall what was said or done—or what wasn't. Then, let it go, without bitterness. It's all in the past, after all, and you are alive today. You may want to do something ritualistic, like burning the piece of paper. Take care of those old memories, so you can set about making new, positive ones.

6 Body Balance

Good Stuff to Support Your Health

As you set about striking a mental and spiritual balance, your eating habits will likely change. Let's make sure that they serve to support your body's daily needs, so that nutritional deficiencies do not drain your immune system. At the same time, you can create the proper internal environment to maintain normal, healthy cell growth in your breasts and the rest of your body.

The human body requires a very specific chemical balance to achieve homeostasis and perform its duties. What you eat and drink either helps or detracts from this balancing act. For instance, cells thrive in somewhat alkaline conditions, at a pH of between 7.0 and 7.4. The standard American diet emphasizes refined sugar and simple carbohydrates, which create a more acidic internal environment that is far from the ideal.

Find out what's going on inside you. Test yourself once or twice a week. You can purchase pH test strips to test saliva or urine for about ten bucks.

The more acidic your blood is, the less oxygen can be absorbed by the red bloods cells in your bloodstream. Likewise, in very acidic states, cells are less able to absorb oxygen from the bloodstream. This is cancer's playground! Unlike normal cells, cancer cells can live long and prosper in a low-oxygen environment. In the interest of avoiding breast cancer and achieving optimum health, then, you should prevent oxidative stress on your body and maintain an alkaline pH.

How can you do that? Here a few ways:

- Manage stress.
- Don't smoke.
- Don't wear tight clothing.
- Drink pure or purified water.
- Adopt an alkaline diet.

The stress response increases body acidity, which lowers the oxygen-carrying capacity of the hemoglobin in your blood. Which cells thrive in low-oxygen conditions? Cancer cells! We have discussed how smoking and wearing tight brassieres restrict blood circulation and deprive the cells of oxygen, making both habits risk factors for breast cancer. We'll talk more about the detriments of bras in Chapter 7; right now, let's concentrate on what you're putting *into* your body to control acidity: liquid, food, and supplements.

***

Good to know . . .

Acids, molecules that form hydronium ions when dissolved in water.
Alkalis, molecules that form hydroxide ions when dissolved in water.
Acid-alkaline balance, the balance between the amount of acids and alkalis in the body necessary to maintain health and homeostasis.

Drink Well (or Well Water!)

Clean water from a quality source is alkaline, just like your body's internal "sea." Whatever else you drink, water should make up a large part of your daily liquid diet. But, as we've seen, city treatment plants and pipelines affect the properties of good, old H_2O. Chlorine additives address the bacteria from animal and human waste that seeps into a water source but do not eliminate heavy metals, chemicals, pesticides, drugs, and other contaminants.

Not all of us are lucky enough to have access to well water from a deep aquifer, probably the most reliable source of the good stuff. If you can't get that, should you be drinking bottled water, then? Not really. That's a Band-Aid that rips open a new wound—those plastic water bottles may pose health threats of their own. "Bad" plastic contains toxic phthalates and bisphenol A (BPA), which are known carcinogens and have been linked with breast cancer. And the water that plastic bottles contain may be nothing but ordinary tap water! Regulatory loopholes can allow this stuff to wind up in your store, labeled as "spring water" or "purified water." Unless *you* know the source, don't trust it.

If you wonder about what's coming out of your faucets, have your water tested. Private and county-sponsored testing services can identify how pure your water is, or isn't. You can also buy digital water pH testers for about $20. If you're already sure that the source is compromised—say, your water comes from a river downstream from major factories, or one into which human sewage backs up during heavy rains . . . or just about any major metropolitan area's source—purify it yourself.

Water filtration systems for the home run about $800 and up, but they protect taps in the whole house, including showers and washing machines. You don't drink out of those? Well, no, you don't; but your skin does. Bathing in or wearing clothes that have been washed in unfiltered water exposes your body's largest organ—your skin—to all of the free-radical chlorine, fluoride, and other chemicals in tap water. As I mentioned, skin's absorptive ability is extremely powerful and quick. If you are cleansing your body in an unfiltered shower, you are absorbing serious amounts of this stuff.

If you can't afford a whole-house system, or if you live in an apartment, shop for under-the-sink models or, at the very least, shower filters that affix to your shower heads. Still saving up? Opt for plastic pitcher-style filters, and pour the treated water into a glass container once it's ready to drink. Anything is better than nothing.

While we're on the subject, take care in how you transport your to-go water as you set out on your busy day. Glass makes the best material for water storage, as it's inert and won't add anything to your drinking water. If you must choose plastic, look for polyethylene bottles labeled #2 or #4 HDPE, which have not been proven to leach chemicals that cause illness.

In selecting your beverages, as well as foods, you'll want a balance between those that are *alkalizing*, or which contribute to an alkaline pH, and those that are *acidifying*, or which create an acidic pH in your body. Try for a ratio of 75 percent alkalizing to 25 percent acidifying. For a full list of these foods and beverages, get one of *The pH Miracle* diet books by nutritionist Dr. Robert Young, or visit a natural medicine Web site.

Here are some examples in the liquid category:

Alkalizing Beverages

Good-quality water
Mineral water
Unpasteurized organic milk
Green tea
Kombucha
Fresh fruit and vegetable juices

Acidifying Beverages

Pasteurized milk (nonorganic)
Rice, soy, and almond milks
Coffee
Beer
Wine
Spirits

You'll notice that I don't list soda, which has no value for your health whatsoever. Now, take a closer look at the second list. If you drink a lot of coffee or alcohol—or much water that contains acidic toxins—you are both tipping your pH balance in the wrong direction and dehydrating your body. "But, I'm not thirsty!" you might argue. That does not mean that your system is properly hydrated. Thirst is actually a *late* physical sign of dehydration; it's just more noticeable than feelings of fatigue, dry skin, and body aches that set in first.

If you're a runner or just aware of fitness trends, you've probably heard that staying hydrated is critical to physical performance. Athletic companies even sell hydration "kits," water receptacles that you strap to your body on long runs or hikes so that you can take sips and avoid dehydration. The human body naturally loses an average of three and a half quarts of water daily, through breathing, excreting urine and feces, and sweat. So if you're sweating buckets, you need to replace that moisture, as well as the electrolytes dissolved in body fluid. You can add one-quarter teaspoon of good salt per quart of water, to help restore electrolyte balance.

So, how much water do you need? Public awareness over this matter has definitely grown. The magic number of 64 ounces per day that is usually tossed around is a good guideline, but the actual amount should be tied to your weight. One ounce of water for every two pounds of body weight should keep you at optimum levels.

Ideally, your body should have all of the water it needs to perform all of its contributions to homeostasis. When you don't provide the water—and food and air—that your body needs to work properly, you invite disease. Chronic dehydration is a very common problem in our culture, with its highly acidic diet and poor-quality water supply. It's easy to tell if you suffer from this problem. If your urine is frequently orange or dark in color, you do. Healthy, hydrated bodies excrete clear urine; those that are slightly dehydrated pass bright yellow urine.

Think of chronic dehydration like chronic stress: it builds up, exacerbating what would otherwise be a minor hiccup in your system. The worse it gets, the greater your chances of experiencing ill consequences. Without enough water, your body cannot flush away the toxins that you ingest, and you already know that toxic buildup attracts cancer growth. So, both the quantity and the quality of the water you drink can protect your breasts and overall health. Be sure to drink often, and drink well!

Eat for Wellness

It's easy to understand the benefits of an alkaline diet if you have already experienced the opposite. Do you need to shift the balance in your daily menus? Your body will tell you. These are symptoms brought on by too many acid-causing foods and drinks:

- Headaches
- Nervousness
- Low energy
- Muscle, joint, or nerve pain or numbness
- Leg cramps
- Nasal congestion
- Excessive mucus production
- Recurring flus, colds, or infections
- Hives and other allergy symptoms
- Indigestion
- Dry skin or hair
- Weak fingernails and toenails
- Development of cysts in the breasts or ovaries

In isolated incidents, these symptoms may be indicative of other medical conditions. If they keep cropping up, purchase those pH test strips to see if your body chemistry is too acidic.

To amend an imbalance or maintain a greater alkaline ratio, what should you eat? Most types of fruits and vegetables and many types of protein foods top the list. It's important to note that **foods that are acidic themselves—such as tomatoes and lemons—may have an alkalizing effect** when subjected to your body's digestive process.

I believe that a variable in your food choices is whether they come from organic or conventional farms. Meat and dairy products from animals that have eaten GMO grains (containing genetically modified organisms) and that have been treated with antibiotics and hormones are acidifying. Their organic counterparts are less so, or not at all. Experiment with your diet, test your pH, and see what you come up with. You may be able to eat more supposedly acid-causing foods without harm if they come from organic sources that minimize that reaction.

Here are some examples of conventionally farmed or raised foods and how they affect you:

Alkalizing Foods

Leafy greens
Root and bulb vegetables
Cruciferous vegetables
Mushrooms
Most fruits
Eggs
Chicken breast meat
Whey protein powder
Cottage cheese
Fermented tofu and tempeh
Almonds and chestnuts
Flax, squash, and sunflower seeds

Acidifying Foods

Most meats and fish
Milk, butter, and most cheeses
Grains
Potatoes
Cranberries
Peas, beans, and peanuts
Brazil nuts, cashews, and pecans
Vegetable, fruit, and seed oils

Again, experiment by choosing organic ingredients or items off the master lists from pH-based dietary references. Test your pH, and watch how your body responds to certain foods.

Additional items that affect your body chemistry include sweeteners, spices, and seasonings. Among these, be sure to eat more salt. One of the many things that physicians have told us that are just dead wrong is to restrict salt. Salt is the essence of life. It contains the basic minerals that allow every nerve, every muscle—indeed, every cell—in the body to function.

So what should your salt look like? Table salt? Absolutely not. Sterile salt is of little value. You want to use salt that still has dozens of natural trace minerals—the kind of nutrients that table salt *used to* contain before it was "refined." You can use sea salt, Himalayan salt, or Real Salt, a brand of salt drawn from mineral-rich deposits in Utah. I personally prefer the Real Salt, which has about sixty trace minerals in it.

All culinary herbs and many spices, such as curry, ginger, black pepper, and turmeric, have healing properties. Use them with confidence. Sweeteners, however, deserve close attention, particularly for women who wish to avoid breast cancer. Be aware that food and beverage labels like to hide sugar under names like maltodextrin, dextrose, fructose and others.

In addition to promoting weight gain, processed sweeteners, such as cane sugar and corn syrup—and foods like white bread and pasta that are high in simple carbohydrates—create acidity, which cancer cells enjoy. More importantly, these items break down easily into glucose molecules. Glucose provides a ready source of energy for voracious cancer cells that need fuel for rapid division and to sustain their prolonged life cycles. Reduce that nutrient, and you can literally starve cancer cells.

Another key nutrient that can tip your healthy dietary balance is fat. The animal, fruit, seed, and vegetable fats that we eat carry the same calorie loads—about 100 calories per tablespoon—but have vastly different effects on the body, some good and some bad. Additionally, dairy butter tends to be overconsumed and contribute to weight gain. In the context of preventing breast cancer and overall body health, the best dietary fats are unsaturated fats that contain Omega-3 fatty acids, followed by those with Omega-6 fatty acids; the least desirable are synthetic trans fats and animal-derived saturated fats.

To give your body the "good" fats it needs, start with cold-water fish like salmon, tuna, and sardines. A consistent intake of fish oil has been shown to reduce the risk of breast cancer. Findings by the Fred Hutchinson Cancer Research Center suggested as much as 32 percent reduction in breast cancer rates among women who took fish oil supplements. I recommend eating oily fish as a healthy protein source one or two times per week, in addition to supplementation.

More sources of good fat include coconut oil, olive oil, avocados, and almonds. Bad fat sources to steer clear of include fatty meats and lard, which are high in saturated fat, and some margarines and hydrogenated vegetable oil, like Crisco' which contain unhealthy trans fat. The FDA allows labels to declare zero trans fat if the content is less than 0.5 grams per serving. That's **not** zero! Canola oil is also a product that claims to be healthy but is produced by irradiating rapeseed, the type of mustard seed from which it is produced. This stuff is not digestible by humans.

Whatever you eat, watch your portion sizes and get a wide variety of alkalizing foods. This will help you naturally manage your weight and build a good nutritional profile. Doing so reduces your breast cancer risk and supports immune system function. This means that your diet is a very powerful tool in health maintenance over which you have great control. Use it!

Do not think, by the way, that weight management doesn't apply to you. Let's do the numbers, ladies. If you are forty years old and you say to yourself, "I only put on two pounds this year," it doesn't sound so bad. But, it adds up. Let's say you are going to live to be ninety years old. Two times fifty is 100 pounds. If you are 140 pounds now, that means you're headed for 240 pounds. Yikes! Believe this: the scale is your friend. Weigh yourself daily, and if you're at a good weight, stay there. If you are overweight, begin to lose two to four pounds a year until you get to your ideal weight as the result of a healthy diet. No "dieting" allowed!

Carrying a lot of extra pounds makes you twice as likely to develop breast cancer. The reason may be, in part, that heavy people tend to eat more acidifying foods and are less likely to exercise. Researchers studying obesity have also determined that overweight women have higher estrogen levels than women of normal weight. These factors will definitely "tip the scales" toward a cancer-friendly environment.

Supplement for Balance

Unless you amend your soil and grow your own food, you are probably not getting the optimal amount of all the nutrients that support your body processes. A trip to the grocery store will not supply everything you need! Google a good nutritional guide online and study it to learn what your diet might not be providing. Because your vitamin and mineral intake will fluctuate if you are eating a rotating variety of foods, as you should, be sure to take a high-quality multivitamin daily. Find one that goes way beyond the recommended daily allowance of important nutrients; it will state the percentage on the label. Consistent levels of the antioxidant vitamins A, C, and E are essential to immune system health.

Some nutritional supplements specifically address the condition of your breasts and ward off cancer. For instance, most cancer patients are hypothyroid, so I always prescribe adequate daily iodine to offset this condition. You can learn more about the science behind them online or in my book, *The Secret of Health: Breast Wisdom*. These include:

- Alpha lipoic acid, a powerful antioxidant
- Calcium d-glucarate, an easily absorbable form of calcium
- Indole-3 caribinol (I3C), a compound that helps regulate estrogen activity
- Iodine, as liquid rubbed into the skin or as iodoral tablets
- Phosphatidylcholine, a nutrient beneficial to immune function
- Probiotics, "good" bacteria, such as acidophilus, that assists digestion
- Red wine extract, another powerful antioxidant
- Vitamin C (at least 4,000mg/day)
- Vitamin D3, or cholecalciferol (20,000IU/day), the best source for Vitamin D
- Vitamin K as M K 7 (100mcg/day)

7 Bras Aren't Wonder-ful

How Bra Wearing Affects Breast Cancer Risk

Fashion is insidious. It entices the wearer and the watcher. Its continual changes make it something to pursue, season in and season out. It has become so entrenched in our market-driven, capitalist culture that many people never question its significance . . . or its impact on health. We look back on the days of corsets and bound feet and chuckle, thinking that disfiguring fashion is a thing of that past. Think again! If you've been wearing a brassiere since your preteen days, your complicity with the fashion industry may be setting you up for health problems.

The topic of dangerous underwear is amusing to some people, but it's no laughing matter. Research has definitively linked bra-wearing habits to breast cancer and other maladies. Surprised? If you're like most Western women, you probably are. You might never have questioned the need to cover and/or support your breasts. The practice is an accepted convention in many cultures, based on social values and lifestyle considerations.

Brassieres were invented, however, before we knew much about breast health. Perhaps bras won't always be in vogue—at least, not in their present design. As women become aware of the dangers of wearing them, they will demand healthier alternatives. Consider how the corset fell out of favor after researchers blamed it for distorting women's spines and causing organ damage. Yes, we still have girdles, bras, and many other body-altering items. Do some research for yourself to see what is behind their continued popularity—it's not just fashion.

If you look online or in the lingerie departments of stores (don't worry, I usually don't!), the array of body-shaping underwear for women shows what a huge gold mine the lingerie business is. In the United States alone, estimated retail bra sales totaled $6.5 billion in 2014. Dozens of bra styles tell women that they should enhance this or minimize that. The message is that something is wrong with them.

Capitalizing on women's insecurity is a time-honored tradition. The cosmetics and cosmetic surgery markets come to mind. But the tide may be turning as priorities shift. *Comfort* is no longer a dirty word for clothing shoppers to use—look at shoe styles and "casual Friday" office trends. Customer demand has pushed beauty products manufacturers to use healthier and organic ingredients in place of harmful ones. In fact, this is an ideal time to consider—perhaps for the first time in your life—whether your bra's benefits outweigh the risks.

***

Good to know . . .

Lymph, body fluid that exists between cells and contains waste products and unused nutrients.

Lymph nodes, oval-shaped organs distributed throughout the lymph vessels, which detect viruses, fungi, and bacteria, and produce antibodies against them.

Lymph vessels, vascular-like tubes that carry lymph away from cells and return it to blood circulation.

Your Bra Is Not a Phone Holder

Maybe it's the *out of sight, out of mind* thing, but women typically give little notice to the issues surrounding bra use. If you were like many other girls, you probably looked forward to getting your first bra and figured it was a matter of *when*, not *if*. Now that you're mature, you may or may not consider this article of clothing optional. I'm not asking you to burn your Wonderbra. I am asking you to look back on your relationship with bras and question its foundations—pardon the pun. Here's a quiz.

1. Do you:

    a) wear a bra every day, without question? For how long?
    b) wear a bra around the clock—even to bed?
    c) peel off your bra as soon as you get home from work?

2. Does your bra:

    a) augment your breasts with padding?
    b) immobilize your breasts?
    c) leave red marks on your body?

3. Is the primary reason for wearing your bra:

    a) for ease of nursing your child?
    b) to make sports activities and movement easier?
    c) to make your breasts more or less noticeable?

Your answers reveal how and why you wear a bra, and whether it is the type most likely to detract from breast health. We learned much about these things through the inquiry of two applied medical anthropologists, Sydney Ross Singer and Soma Grismaijer, who between 1991 and 1993 surveyed the bra-wearing attitudes and habits of 4,700 women, many of whom had breast cancer. Here are some statistics from their study that will shed light on your answers to question 1:

- Women who wear bras for more than 12 hours per day have a 1 in 7 chance of getting breast cancer; this rises to a 3 in 4 chance with 24-hour bra use.
- Women who wear bras for less than 12 hours per day have a 1 in 152 chance.
- Women who rarely or never wear a bra have a 1 in 168 chance.

The researchers determined that factors relating to dress *do* influence the rate of disease. Most importantly, they found a 125-fold difference in the incidence of breast cancer between women who never wore bras and those who never took theirs off. In other words, wearing a bra twenty-four hours a day catapults cancer risk. Singer and Grismaijer published their findings in the book *Dressed to Kill: the Link Between Breast Cancer and Bras*, inviting other researchers to replicate or expand on their work in a controlled study.

You don't see scientists jumping to do this—maybe because the bra industry isn't about to fund this kind of research. Besides, Singer and Grismaijer received blatant death threats over this research and publication. While the topic remains controversial, as a physician and practicing oncologist, I can attest that **bras do, indeed, play a role in the development of breast cancer.** Let's consider how physical effects of wearing a bra could do so.

In question 2, if you acknowledged wearing a padded bra, your garment increases the temperature of your breasts. If you said you wear a very firm support bra that restricts or eliminates breast movement, your lingerie restricts lymphatic circulation in the area. Red marks left on your body after you remove your bra indicate constriction that affects blood circulation to the breasts, chest, and shoulders—not to mention restricting the flow of *chi*, the life force or energy flow, according to the Chinese culture.

If you suffer from these or other effects, you'll want to examine why you wear a bra in the first place. Is it to facilitate nursing, the purpose for which your breasts are designed? Is it for practical reasons, to manage a heavy bust or for comfort during vigorous activity? Or, is it to conceal or reveal your breasts, as social situations dictate? Your answers to question 3 display your motivation for putting on an undergarment, which may or may not be comfortable, as often as you do.

Now that Pandora's box is open, let's look at the mechanics of what is really going on when you fasten those hooks.

The Smoking Gun

Bras, although loaded by society with sexual meaning, are not meant as weapons to be used against their wearers—unless it's to create emotional pressure to purchase them. The strain of trying to live up to contrived standards of beauty that have no bearing on the true shape or purpose of breasts may have health implications all its own. But we are concerned with the more evident physical changes that take place when wearing them—some of which create the special conditions that cancer cells prefer.

Let's start with temperature. The position of the breasts as an appendage slightly removed from the body's core means that their normal temperature is a degree or two cooler than the usual 98.6 degrees. The breasts are designed this way because they function optimally at that lower temperature. Covering them traps body heat and raises their temperature. Bras are close-fitting, so their insulating properties are significant.

Increased temperature in the breasts may affect hormonal action in their vicinity. Since we know that cancer cells are attracted to elevated temperatures, and that estrogen plays a role in breast cancer's development, messing with that equation could well invite disease.

Another tantalizing environment for cancer is one that is low in oxygen. Reducing blood flow to the breast area satisfies that requirement! Bras are made with elastic bands to grab the torso and squeeze, forming a foundation from which to lift the breasts. Shoulder straps are also elasticized, and supporting the weight of heavy breasts tightens those straps against the body. If you see red marks that outline your bra after you take it off, it's impacting the oxygen level in your breast tissue. Restricting blood circulation also slows the delivery of nutrients to breast cells, which you want to remain as robust as possible.

Bra design also affects lymphatic flow, the process that carries toxins away from cells. Bras that come up under your armpits put pressure on the many lymph nodes there. Bras that keep your breasts from moving naturally—this would be most bras, but especially those with underwire support—greatly restrict lymphatic and *chi* circulation. Since lymph vessels do not expand and contract as the heart pumps, the way blood vessels do, periodic physical movement is needed to push the lymph along. While breathing and shifting weight effect this in other parts of the body, the breasts are meant to move with body motion, especially walking.

Singer and Grismaijer believe that **the presence of toxins brought on by poor lymph drainage is one cause of breast cancer**. If your lymph nodes and vessels near your breasts are "stopped up," toxins will accumulate there, potentially to alarming levels, if the situation is never relieved. Efficient lymph drainage is essential to immune system health, and is therefore critical to guarding against or healing breast cancer.

Dress Accordingly

So, you've worn a bra for your entire adult life; now what? As with adopting any new behavior, only you can decide whether the trade-off is worth it. If you conclude that intervention is called for, you can go whole-hog and abandon your bra . . . or take gradual steps toward reducing its effects on your breasts' welfare by wearing it fewer hours each day.

First, return to your answer to question 3, above. Why do you wear a bra? How necessary to your everyday priorities is it? Just thinking about this matter will help you map out a plan. If you wear a bra primarily for social reasons, you can consider not wearing one when you're alone. If you are nursing, you can also change your dress habits when your baby grows past the nursing stage.

Don't think you have to do make radical progress all at once. If you've spent a lifetime encased in a bra, you'll have a lot of emotional baggage around the subject as well. Do some test runs to see how many hours you can comfortably go bra-free, or during which activities. Maybe you'll lose some of your social inhibitions as time goes by and begin to detach your self-image from others' opinions of your appearance, as far as breast coverage goes.

The bottom line is: you're a big girl now, and you dress yourself. You're informed and can make your own choices. I hope you'll choose health, even if it's by degrees. Here are a couple more tips to make transitioning out of bra bondage easier:

- Avoid underwires.
- Avoid padding; the thinner the material, the less insulating it is to the breasts.
- If you see red marks on your skin, loosen your bra.
- If you can't loosen your bra, it's too small! Get a bra that fits.
- Try wearing a loose camisole or a thin crop top.
- Pick a time of day to "rest" your breasts.
- Don't sleep in your bra!

8 Move It or Lose It

How Exercise Reduces Breast Cancer Risk

When it comes to breast health, there's something to be said for the aphorism, *move it or lose it*. Wearing a more forgiving bra or going without one some or all of the time are two ways to get the breasts moving. *Lymphatic pump,* or the means of transporting lymph fluid, is essential for healthy breasts—so a little bounce is actually necessary. Of course, your whole body must be conditioned if you are to enjoy a long, active life. **Exercising your body also reduces your risk for breast cancer,** so moving it really does prevent losing it.

Some of you are nodding your heads, while others groan. In the modern world in which physical labor and locomotion are frequently optional, fitness is a personal choice. I know of a woman in her mid-fifties who is overweight and just now beginning to show symptoms related to sedentary living. "I'm not the exercise type," she claims—and I get that. We all have lifestyle preferences. But nature doesn't give a hoot about our lifestyles.

Not exercising regularly eventually relieves you of the ability to move without pain. Among other health issues, this workout-averse woman is suffering knee pain from joint deterioration, hastened by her extra weight. She faces surgery and her doctor's dictum to begin no-impact exercise in the meantime. She is still procrastinating. Once you are in pain, starting an exercise program is even more distasteful than it was. But it's better than being partially or permanently disabled!

If you're the "exercise type," that's fantastic. If you're not, I've got just the ticket. It's called motivation. You're reading this book because you care about the health of your breasts and body. Let's take a more in-depth look at the *why* of exercise. Then we'll look at several different *hows*, to either pump up your existing routine or get you started off on the right foot.

***

Good to Know . . .

Aerobic exercise, vigorous physical activity that requires the heart to pump hard enough to supply additional oxygen to meet cellular demand.
Chronic disease, illness such as cancer and diabetes that develops and/ or persists over many years.
Malignancy, an invasive cancerous tumor.

A Body in and out of Motion

Your survival instinct is innate and strong. If you need a reason to become or remain active, how does staying alive longer sound to you? How about extending the life spans of your children, too? Mounting scientific evidence regarding exercise benefits has brought greater public awareness to the issue. How much and what kind of exercise is best, and the effects of routine physical activity, have now been documented; so, no waffling! The first conclusion to take to heart is that **some exercise—whatever it is, even for a few minutes a day—is better than none.**

Regularly exercising reduces your chances of developing chronic disease, which is the top killer worldwide. In the United States, heart disease, cancer (all types), and respiratory disease are the three leading causes of death. Your risk for all of these conditions falls if you exercise for about thirty minutes on most days of the week. If you keep moving and eat right, you can also prevent or delay the onset of type 2 diabetes, osteoporosis, and osteoarthritis, which all have painful, debilitating, or life-threatening side effects.

Not only has exercise been shown to prevent chronic diseases, a *lack of exercise* has been revealed as a primary *cause* of them. So, researchers have closed the loop. Furthermore, long-term illnesses such as high blood pressure and type 2 diabetes that were once the domain of older Americans are now showing up in youngsters, largely due to a poor diet and sedentary lifestyle. Estimates in 2012 projected that more than one-third of Americans under age twenty were overweight. Because adults set examples for children, it's no wonder that kids whose parents are overweight are 80 percent more likely to become overweight than children of normal-weight parents. So, we pass along our problems to the next generation. It doesn't have to be that way.

The benefits of physical fitness appear in studies that show a decline in the rate of chronic diseases and premature death among those who get with the program. If you need another reason to work out other than avoiding an early demise, consider the cost of long-term illness. It's a financial killer, with unending expenses: ambulance trips, doctor and hospital bills, prescription drugs, time lost from work . . . the list goes on and on.

Multiple mental health studies have also revealed that exercise prevents and treats depression, another negative influence on your physical condition. All chronic diseases place stress on the immune system, and that, we have learned, is a contributing factor for breast cancer. So, changing sedentary to more active habits holds many consequences for breast health.

What are the magic numbers associated with working out? Accumulated research shows that performing moderate-intensity activity (such as brisk walking) in increments that total two and a half hours per week optimizes brain and heart function. Less is still helpful; more is even better. But you need to work out safely and not overdo it to start with.

We'll talk about how regular walks around the block or trips to the gym specifically affect your breast health in a minute. What's important right now is your *why*. Consider embracing these motivators—and add your personal favorites to the list:

Top 3 Reasons to Work Out

1. Longer, healthier life
2. Bigger bank account
3. Looking your best

Why Cancer Adores Couch Potatoes

We've touched on all of the reasons why exercise helps and sedentary behavior harms breast health, but let's tie those threads together. Assume that if you exercise, you're more likely to maintain good cardiovascular condition and a reasonable weight. That's a good thing.

Excess weight increases breast cancer risk for older women, partly because it results in undue estrogen production, which invites cancer to settle in the breasts. Remember, the breasts are mostly made of fat. Recall, also, that estrogen is made by the ovaries and by fat cells. Before menopause, the ovaries produce the majority of estrogen; after menopause, fat cells do. This is why the breasts are a prime cancer target overall. Heavy women have more fat tissue, so they produce more estrogen, and their breast cancer risk is increased.

Excess weight is a concern for younger women because, barring a change of lifestyle, they will go on to add to their body mass, especially when their metabolism changes in midlife. They are also more susceptible to inflammatory breast cancer, the most aggressive form of malignancy in the breasts, which tends to appear in premenopausal women at a higher rate than other forms of breast cancer. Inflammatory breast cancer is more common in obese women than those of normal weight.

The less you exercise, the more likely you are to have high blood sugar and low blood oxygen. Although high blood sugar, or glucose, is related to your eating habits, it is an invitation to cancer to come on over and watch TV with you. Maintaining little oxygen in tissue is like handing cancer cells the channel changer. And, sitting idle also restricts lymph flow and allows toxins to build up in the body. This is the equivalent of free popcorn.

The more you exercise, though, the more likely you are to have active lymph drainage, normal blood sugar—and normal blood oxygen levels.

Aerobic exercise increases your heart rate and blood circulation, sending more nutrients and oxygen, as well as the white blood cells that kill cancer, to all your cells. When you move, you stimulate the lymphatic system as well, helping to flush toxins from the body and improve your immune response. If you want to end your unhealthy relationship with cancer and retain healthy and intact breasts, get up off the couch! Here's how.

Just Love It

Sorry, Nike: just doing it is not enough. Like sticking to a healthy diet, committing to exercise takes more than just liking a sport or social hour at the gym. If you're going to incorporate an activity into the rest of your life, you had better love it.

You have enough obligations. Don't make working out a chore. Do you love the outdoors? Get out there and ride a horse or a bike, play tennis or soccer, run or walk. You're not outdoorsy? There are indoor tennis courts and soccer grids, or you might enjoy the more structured atmosphere of the fitness center. Swimming is an excellent non-weight-bearing choice, especially if you have musculoskeletal problems. If you're social, take an exercise or dance class. If you're not, practice yoga or work out on a machine at home.

Mix it up, so you work different muscle groups and don't get bored. If you were to make a list of all the different ways to expend energy, you'd be bound to find one that strikes your fancy. And what about the things that you'd rather not do but that still burn calories and make your blood pump? Yard work, housework, and climbing stairs all count as exercise.

For total body fitness, you want to include aerobics, muscle building, and bone strengthening. Some activities, like gardening, fulfill all those objectives. Do not try to "get it over with" by doing two or three solid hours of any exercise, though. You don't want to strain a muscle or get physically or mentally burned out. I recently saw some good advice that suggested exercising to 50 percent of your capacity—in duration and intensity. You'll find out as you go along what makes your body happy and when you've crossed the line. Whether you exercise first thing in the morning, over your lunch break, or after work, aim for a well-rounded session that warms you up, cools you down, and places good stress on your heart in between.

To make sure I don't run out of time to exercise—a prime excuse for anyone—I put in thirty minutes soon after I roll out of bed every morning. I cover all my bases by doing 50 push-ups, 30 jumping jacks, and a few sets of leg pumps on my Xciser, making sure to raise my heart rate to 150 three times during my routine. I include 10 pull-ups, 20 sit-ups, and some lifts with hand weights to condition my upper torso and arms. Because I travel a lot, it helps to have a routine that I can practice anywhere. I add other enjoyable activities, like hiking and skiing, as my schedule allows. I used to be extremely active with outdoor sports, but as my kids grew up, the pace of my life changed; so I have practiced my present regimen for the last ten years.

Do you need to buy machines, gadgets, health club memberships, or special workout clothing to exercise? Of course not. But if those things keep you motivated, go for it. After your routine has become a routine, the long-term benefits are what will keep you going. You'll notice that you feel better when you exercise, and crave a workout when you don't. And when the subject of breast cancer prevention pops up on the news or online, you can check *regular exercise* off your list—and feel great about it.

9 The Detox Challenge

How to Relieve Toxic Effects on the Body

Now that your circulation is optimized and you're putting wonderful stuff into your body, let's take purification to the next level. You've been mulling over your choices in reducing or avoiding contact with the toxins around you. Let's turn your decisions into action.

In Chapter 3, I waved some major warning flags to show you how important it is for you to take charge of the things in your life and your environment that can invite cancer to inhabit your body. Next, I'll give you some tips for how to get started doing that. Consider detoxification, like exercise, a lifelong habit to pursue. It seems that as soon as one environmental health problem is solved, two more take its place. Don't give in! Your life depends on it.

Again, break down your intentions into three groups: begin to address things that have a toxic effect on your person, your household, and the rest of the wide world in which you live. You don't have to do it all at once. Read some labels, sort through your belongings for questionable items, and—most importantly—listen to your inner knower as you make your daily choices. If you sense that something is dragging you down, it probably is.

***

Good to Know . . .

Antibody, a protein used by the immune system to eliminate harmful antigens.

Antigen, a molecule that provokes an immune response, which often resides within foreign substances that enter the body, such as bacteria, fungi, and viruses.

Autism, a neurological condition that affects how the brain processes information.

Carcinogenic, cancer causing.

Electromagnetic field, an electric charge in the immediate atmosphere caused by an electrical signal from cell phones, radios, televisions, microwaves, and house wiring.

Your Body, Your Self

Let's return to your first home—the palace that is your body, mind, and spirit. You may already use a variety of "natural" soap, hair care, and cosmetic items that you consciously chose for their health value. Meanwhile, many other personal products that you take for granted are exposing you to poisonous ingredients, sometimes several times a day. Chemicals and other junk you don't need hide behind innocuous or scientific-sounding names on product labels—even the ones that you think are natural.

It's not your fault. Marketing is a cruel thing, especially when it comes to promoting products that directly affect your body. Government regulation is weak at best, with the USDA having rendered the term *organic* nearly meaningless. But at least food products have to meet some specifications; personal care products can be billed as organic with absolutely no basis for the claim.

Consider that your skin absorbs certain topical ingredients directly into your bloodstream. That stuff is circulating around in there every day, with elements that your body can't use piling up in its filtering system, your liver. I'll show you how to detoxify your liver at the end of this chapter. But, why not head this petrochemical army off at the pass? Do some research on natural and synthetic ingredients common to body and clothing care products, so you can distinguish pure from poison. You can look online at natural health and green living Web sites to find a comprehensive list of personal care ingredients. Meanwhile, gather your containers and analyze the laundry detergent, cleansers, cosmetics, and other things you buy that come in contact with your skin and hair on a regular basis.

Keep the healthy ones, and banish the rest! Remove the ones with the following compounds that are known to cause cancer and/or harm the immune system:

Toxic Chemicals to Watch Out For

Formaldehyde. This carcinogenic gas can dissolve in liquids and enter the body through the skin, or it can be ingested from the air. In 2015, manufacturer Johnson & Johnson admitted using this toxic ingredient in baby shampoo and other items. The company later paid $72 million in damages to the family of a woman who died of ovarian cancer that was linked to her daily use of its talcum powder products, but it was too late.

Formaldehyde might be listed on label ingredients, or it can hide amid other compounds called formaldehyde-releasing preservatives (FRPs) that emit formaldehyde gas when they break down. Steer clear of anything containing polyoxyethylene or ingredients that include "PEG," "eth," or "oxynol" in their names.

Formaldehyde ingredients are commonly found in hair and nail care products, mascara, and makeup removers; check shampoos and cosmetics!

1,4-dioxane. Here's another known carcinogen that travels incognito in products like laundry soap, makeup, and other personal care items. It might not make the product labels because it's not "added" but is formed during manufacturing. Dioxane (not the same as *dioxin*) hides within well-known ingredients like sodium laureth sulfate. In 2010, dangerous levels of the chemical were found in what would seem to be a "healthy" line of hair products, Herbal Essences, made by Proctor and Gamble.

I'd like to tell you to check your laundry detergents, but perhaps you should write to your congressperson, instead. Both China and the United States do not yet regulate this dangerous chemical.

Triclosan. This ingredient present in antibacterial and antimicrobial soaps, wipes, and toothpastes may cause liver cancer, as reported in 2014 in *Proceedings of the National Academy of Sciences*. The chemical was developed for use in surgical scrubs but is now prevalent in a slew of personal care products.

Cumulative research on the widespread use of antibacterials in general suggests that long-term exposure can make bacteria resistant to the antibiotics meant to kill them. So, these products are worse than useless! The 2014 study indicates that triclosan damages human livers, making it even more difficult to rid yourself of toxins. That's bad news for your immune system.

Even more ominous to women concerned about breast cancer, further research suggests that triclosan interferes with thyroid hormone uptake and may affect other hormonal processes. The truth is, your body is designed to kill bacteria, and you don't want it to lose that ability. Get rid of antibacterial stuff; check your soap!

Paint It Green

All of the above chemicals can be found in some household cleaners and building and decorating materials, such as carpeting, fiberboard, synthetic flooring, paints, and varnishes. There's a good reason why many honchos in the construction industry have embraced green technology—their employees were getting sick and dying.

It's time that household cleaning manufacturers stepped up to the plate to reduce their customers' risk—largely borne by women—for developing cancer. A 2010 study found that among a group of 1,500 women, those with the most frequent use of household cleaning products were 50 percent more likely to get a diagnosis of breast cancer than women who used those products the least.

You have a choice in what you use to mop up spills or get gunk off fixtures. Although federal regulations may be spotty, makers of products that have certain levels of toxicity have to warn you about them on the labels. You women who do the cleaning in your houses might find it ironic that these legal warning definitions are based on the effects of a 180-pound man inhaling, swallowing, or absorbing these poisons through the skin. Go ahead and extrapolate your own risk—and that of your children! Here's what those warnings mean:

How Toxic Is "Toxic"?

- **Caution.** One ounce to one pint (and up) of the substance may be harmful or fatal.
- **Warning.** One teaspoon to one ounce (or more) may be harmful or fatal.
- **Danger.** A "taste" to one teaspoon (at least) *is definitely* fatal.

We're all leery of skull-and-crossbones–type chemicals getting into our systems and making us sick. But what about the other things in household air that you can't see? I'm talking about the electromagnetic fields (EMFs) radiated by the dozens of electrical appliances in your home.

Research in the U.S. suggests but has yet to prove that EMFs can cause cancer, but the possibility is widely accepted. Research in Europe shows a definitive association, so leaders took quick action to protect children, whose developing bodies are most vulnerable. The Council of Europe advises member nations to avoid health risks by banning cell phones and wireless internet connections from schools.

If this type of radiation *is* a problem, the consequences could be very far reaching, given the pervasiveness of EMF sources in the environment. Everything from high-voltage power lines to wireless electronics—including cell phones—tosses this radiation into the atmosphere around you. Remember: your bra is not a cell phone holder! Never ever, ever put your cell in your bra.

We've discussed microwave ovens, which are big culprits due to their enormous power draw and EMF output. If you must use these and other electrical appliances, you can reduce your EMF exposure by simply standing back while they function. That's fine during the daytime. You should take special care at night, though. During sleep, your brain directs special rejuvenating functions in your body that could be upset by electromagnetic radiation. EMFs emit signals that confuse your neuro-immune system and prevent it from functioning properly. Be sure to keep a buffer zone around your bed—and especially, your head—while you sleep. That means, no cell phones, clocks, aromatherapy machines, fans, or other appliances in close proximity to your brain.

Scheduled for Removal

You can take all the precautions you like, there will still be negative influences on your breasts and body that you can't control. To those things, you must say, "Out! Out, damned spot!" Detoxification of the colon and liver is one way of going about this. Avoiding conventional medical doctors is another. I'll tell you why.

Medical science has been inextricably tied to the federal government, Big Pharma, medical supply manufacturers, and insurance companies—all of which have interests in controlling how you receive your health care. Compassion and integrity may be at the bottom of their lists. Then there are the medical providers, themselves. Doctors are people, and people have faults like pride and ignorance that get in the way of what works. Sad but true.

This is why **patients in the conventional health care system are subjected to known dangers, like x-rays, antibiotics, vaccines, and interactive and addictive drugs.** I call the medical professionals who continue to use these treatments willfully ignorant, for they know these things are bad for you and that there are safer healing alternatives. But, either they are in the pocket of one of the Big Guys, or they don't want to be embarrassed by having to admit that what they've done for years was wrong. I would remind them of the Hippocratic oath they took, which says, *first, do no harm.*

Take the case of mammograms: the profitable mammogram industry wants to keep its place at the top of the screening totem pole, regardless of the fact that its service causes cancer, pain, and anxiety in women. Hmm. How do you feel about that?

Here's another example: vaccines, including flu shots. The theory behind them is that they dose the body with killed or weakened viruses to prompt the immune system to form an antibody. These altered viruses mimic the real things. Should the real virus invade the body, theoretically, it recognizes the antigen and attacks and kills it. But how closely are scientists replicating disease-causing viruses? The drug companies have knowingly given us vaccines containing monkey viruses that they knew would cause cancer. Throw in mercury or methimazole, an antithyroid drug—plus too many viruses in a given vaccine for the body to respond to—and you have a toxic cocktail that causes disease and cancer.

That does not lead to immunity! Vaccines do not create immunity. Immunity is what occurs when you get the measles or mumps and your body forms an immune response to them. We now know that vaccines cause autism, and that the Centers for Disease Control and Prevention have tried to cover up this data. Go for natural immunity by pursuing a healthy regimen instead of relying on vaccines. Do yourself a favor and watch the movie *Vaxxed: From Cover-up to Catastrophe.*

Vaccines, antibiotics, and x-rays have been ingrained into medical protocol. Changing entrenched attitudes takes a long time. That means you've got to be your own advocate. You must maintain your health, and you must seek out the best healing options should your health fail. I have some excellent maintenance tips for you in the next chapter—things you can do at home or places where you can find alternative and complementary care. But, sometimes, regular doctors and hospitals can't be avoided. What you can do to reduce their toxic effects on you is to know when to resist their pressure to do the wrong things.

Health care practitioners are an opinionated bunch. They go to school for a long time. They see a lot of patients. They have influence over those patients' very lives, and they're paid to render medical advice. But that's the key—it's *advice*. They cannot tell you what to do. **It is your body, and you alone get to decide what is done to it.**

Still, many patients believe their doctors have the authority to choose for them, or simply that "they must know best." As we've seen, they often do not.

Give yourself the authority to say *no, ma'am,* or even just *maybe,* or *let me think it over; I'll get back to you.* You take the initiative, or the professionals will. Do your homework, listen to your inner knower, and *you* decide whether to submit to:

- Mammograms
- Other x-rays and CT scans
- Antibiotic drugs
- Vaccines

In the interest of cleansing your body from harmful elements that you cannot escape in the environment, you really must learn a few methods of detoxification. These involve helping the digestive system—which is normally charged with this task—to overcome challenges it wasn't designed to handle.

We are inundated with toxins every day. The human liver can only process today's delivery of pollution and poison; whatever it can't filter during that period remains as toxic residue in your system. Even when the liver succeeds in moving unwanted matter through to the intestinal tract, the colon, in doing its job of waste removal, might not detoxify everything. It might be sluggish due to whatever you ate last night, and the leftover toxins and bacteria can build up there, too.

The solutions open to every one of us have been used to purge the body of poison for a long time. They've fallen out of favor because they don't make the drug companies any money. These include fasting, or food abstinence, and colonic irrigation, or enemas.

Fasting, in which you suspend your intake of food, is a lost art in our culture that is obsessed with eating for eating's sake. Fasting cuts off the body's supply of glucose and forces it to use its stores in the muscles and liver for energy. After it eats that up, it turns to fatty tissue. Any toxins hanging out there are dissolved as the fat is "burned." So stay well hydrated with water during a fast to keep flushing the toxins out.

A primary benefit of fasting for breast health is rejuvenation of the immune system. When your body is short on fuel, it tries to conserve energy. One way is for it to jettison senescent immune cells—those that are old or damaged and no longer useful. Your neuro-immune system prompts worn-out white blood cells to die off, making way for new ones to grow. The body does this naturally, of course, but needs help every now and then to restore its efficiency.

Once an active white blood cell has identified something to attack—a virus, bacteria, chemical, fungus, cancer cell, etc.—it is programmed to respond only to that antigen, limiting its range. Fasting allows these cells to die off and lets new ones that can identify other targets grow to take their place. This mechanism is a wonderful aid to healing breast cancer patients, and in particular, those whose immune systems have been wrecked by chemotherapy.

To maintain and refresh immune function, I recommend a 48-hour fast, with water only, at least once a month. You can do it, be you healthy, diabetic, or battling cancer. Again, taking adequate amounts of water is very important. I recommend beginning a fast after lunch on the first day and then ending it by eating dinner on the third day, with a 48-hour spread in between. That way you only go to bed really hungry one night. If you fast for longer periods, you will need to reintroduce food carefully, as your stomach will have shrunk. Begin by eating fruit and simple carbs one evening and the next day adding nuts and cooked vegetables, to build back up to your regular dietary intake.

In addition to fasting, assist your liver and colon in eliminating built-up toxins and bacteria with periodic cleansing. You can do this by visiting a professional colon therapist for colonic irrigation, or by administering a coffee enema yourself. This detoxification technique has been used for hundreds of years, as coffee was known to herbalists to boost the liver. Beginning in the 1920s, coffee enemas were successfully used by Dr. Max Gerson to treat cancer patients for pain and toxicity. I recommend an organic coffee enema at least once weekly to my at-risk patients. If you are taking more than one a week, you'll need to take probiotic supplements to resupply your body with ample "good" bacteria.

Compounds in coffee enemas work to relax the smooth muscles of the colon and dilate blood vessels and bile ducts. This increases bile flow from the liver and gallbladder. Coffee compounds also trigger a flood of the enzyme *glutathione S-transferase (GST)*, which neutralizes free-radical oxygen molecules that would otherwise damage cells. All of the "bad stuff" is dissolved in bile and then excreted through the colon.

Still not convinced? Not so long ago, enemas were a very common home remedy. That was before we had a pill for everything. Once Big Pharma took over our minds, home remedies became discredited. After you get past the postmodern taboos, which arose with the marketing of commercial laxatives, you can take advantage of this simple detox procedure. Don't worry about the effects of caffeine in your bloodstream; if you perform the enema correctly, it goes directly to your liver, and you won't absorb it into your systemic circulation. For a full explanation of coffee enemas, see my Web site: www.drbenmd.com. Here are the basics on how to do it.

A Coffee Enema Cleanse

1. Clear your system with a bowel movement or a plain-water (filtered or distilled) enema.
2. Boil 2 to 3 tablespoons of organic coffee in 2 to 3 cups of filtered water for 5 to 10 minutes.
3. Pour the liquid through a strainer, to remove coffee grounds, and into an enema bag or bucket.
4. Lubricate your anus and the enema tube nozzle with coconut oil.
5. Hang the enema bag or bucket and lie down beneath it.
6. Insert the nozzle into your body, let the liquid flow in, and relax.
7. Hold the solution internally for 15 minutes; then, get up and release it into the toilet.

During the cleanse, you might hear gurgles and feel squirts in your digestive tract, which is perfectly normal. This happens when your gallbladder, which rests beneath your rib cage, empties. If you have trouble retaining the brewed coffee, try the process with smaller volumes of liquid and gradually work up to a full amount. Afterwards, run to the commode, and allow the dissolved toxins to leave your body, along with any anxiety that you may have harbored over the process. You're free!

Notice how you feel afterwards. Any pain that you may have experienced as a result of toxic effects will dissipate or disappear. Your energy level will rise—as will your peace of mind.

PART THREE

10 Education, Not Medication

Oversee Your Health Upkeep Wisely

As you avoid and limit of all the draining influences on your breasts and body, you still must be vigilant in monitoring your health. You're doing a great job! But some matters are out of your hands. Where the breasts are concerned, risk factors such as family history, race, and existing conditions—not to mention your record of past medical interventions—may still enable disease to take hold.

One loophole that hasn't been discussed yet is the importance of refreshing sleep (while *not* encased in a bra!). Quality sleep—continuous sleep that allows you to progress through all the stages, including deep REM sleep—is integral to brain and memory function, hormonal balance, cellular repair, and general immune system R&R. Insomnia or interrupted sleep disrupts these restorative processes.

We have known for a long time that sleep disorders weaken the immune system, but now we know why. A 2012 study conducted in the U.K. and the Netherlands found that prolonged sleeplessness induces the stress response, as evidenced by certain white blood cell activity. Loss of even half a night's sleep alters brain cell function and cuts short the body's release of healing hormones. Higher levels of stress hormones and lower levels of those that help your body fight off the day's toxic effects equal immune system strain that you don't need.

Set yourself up for sleep success by giving your bedroom a healthy makeover. Researchers agree that these elements affect your ability to move through the stages of sleep that allow your body to rejuvenate:

- Mattress and pillow support
- Electromagnetic Fields
- Temperature
- Clutter
- Light
- Noise

Approach each of these factors with your health in mind. In choosing a bed, mattress, and pillows, natural and organic materials that conform to individual needs are musts. These bedding items are typically made from cotton, latex, and/or sheep's wool and are free from toxins that release fumes. Choose those that claim to include organic and unbleached cotton, if possible. Natural latex supports and cradles the spine and neck, while wool helps to regulate body temperature and wick moisture. Air flow beneath your body discourages mold and dust mites. Some healthy mattress/bed combinations, such as the SAMINA sleep system, achieve the ideal combination of support and air flow using safe and natural materials. You'll find many sources for these bedding products online.

We've already talked about keeping electrical appliances away from your bed and head. Sleep experts also note that—even though your eyes are closed—a clutter-free room that is quiet or masks disturbing sounds invites you to drift off and stay asleep. They consider the best temperature for sleep to be an even 65 degrees, so select your bedding and air temperature control to achieve that target year-round.

Light levels can disrupt sleep as well. Turn off the lights in your bedroom at night. What do you see? We have so many appliances and power cords with little lights on them, LED clocks, and outdoor street lights to deal with. See what you can eliminate in your bedroom. The measurement is, when you douse the lights, you shouldn't be able to see your hand in front of your face.

To avoid the threats to your breast and body health, snooze seven to nine hours a night in a healthy environment—free of EMFs and noise pollution, on a bed and bedding that you can trust next to your skin. Who doesn't want more sleep? You'll get it if you put it on your health maintenance list as a priority. As a motivator, SAMINA will honor a discount if you mention the code "Radical Rethink."

Keep immune system health in mind as you build your healthy check-up routine. That means choosing safe and natural breast support procedures, like the no-brainer breast self-exam and breast massage. It also means selecting the least-invasive screening methods, such as thermograms and ultrasounds, and the primary care physicians most likely to share your concerns. Let's pull out the user manual and open up the body shop.

*** *

Good to know . . .

CAM, complementary and alternative medicine, or health care that integrates various modalities, such as the use of vitamins, nutritional herbs, and acupuncture.

Chiropractic, treatment of the musculoskeletal system for related disorders and their effect on general health.

Homeopathy, a health care system that derives remedies for illness based on symptomatic presentation, based on the theory that "like cures like."

Naturopathy, holistic medical care focusing on noninvasive treatment and health maintenance using homeopathy, dietary guidance, herbalism, and other CAM practices.

Your Body Shop

Awareness of what's normal for *your* breasts will allow you to recognize changes and alter the behavior that might invite cancerous growth. Do you feel heat in a breast? Notice changes in shape? Actually find a lump? Again, your inner knower might even hint that something's not quite right. Any of your suspicions are valid, and they can be confirmed or dispelled by getting the right tests (**not** mammograms!) from qualified interpreters. Tests such as thermography can also be used as routine screening to suggest when conditions that *you* can't detect might affect your breast health.

You'll want to pair periodic screening with professional exams and treatments, preferably outside of the conventional medicine community. Alternative care providers such as naturopathic and homeopathic physicians, acupuncturists, chiropractors, and alternative-minded DOs and MDs can provide guidance on all sorts of supportive supplements and therapies. Massage therapy, for instance, has many "trickle-down" health benefits for the breasts. In fact, besides getting regular massage from licensed therapists and exams from medical professionals, you can—and should—DIY.

When young women first go to see a gynecologist or another women's health physician, they are usually tutored and encouraged to perform breast self-examinations (BSEs) on a monthly basis. What's not as common is advice on performing self-massage, to counteract the effects of bra wearing and to stimulate lymphatic flow in the breasts. Years of being bullied by medical doctors into thinking that you aren't qualified to handle your own body may have caused you to avoid looking at or touching your breasts. You should be aware of the value of self-care and understand that it's not only acceptable but preferable to do it!

Consider yourself the proprietor of your own body shop, where you are your best customer. Here's your instruction manual for two important diagnostic and maintenance procedures. You can find video instructions for BSEs on my Web site.

How to Do Breast Self-Exam

I add this here because I've examined at least ten thousand pairs of breasts. I ask my patients if they do their own breast exams, with the answer frequently being yes. I then ask them to demonstrate how they examine themselves . . . it is, indeed, rare when someone comes close to a proper exam.

1. Use a full-length mirror, if possible, to visually check breast appearance. With hands on hips, note their usual color, shape, and size. If one or both breasts look different to you, make a note of:

   • Variations in shape or fullness between the two breasts
   • Skin that bulges, puckers, or dimples
   • Nipple position
   • Any swelling, soreness, or red areas

2. Repeat this inspection with arms raised above your head.
3. Lower your arms and bring them behind your back, watching your nipple movement. Both nipples should move at the same time, in sync with the rest of your body.
4. Lie on your back and place an arm behind your head. With your free hand, explore the tissue of your opposite breast, using the first few fingers in a firm, smooth manner, keeping constant contact with your skin and moving systematically in small circles across the entire surface of your breast. You are feeling for any unusual masses; note that tissue will feel naturally harder or softer in spots, and that's okay. Cover the entire breast area and on over into your armpit as well. Then repeat on the other breast and armpit.
5. Check each nipple for discharge. Start about three inches from the nipple and move toward it, pressing downward with your fingers now, a few times. Then gently squeeze each nipple between your thumb and index finger. Take note of the color of any discharge, which may range from milky white to yellow, slightly bloody, or black. Although the latter could be a sign of a common and harmless fungus, you should share the presence of black or bloody discharge with your physician.
6. Repeat the movements in Step 4 while standing or sitting, examining both breasts once more.

You can put a few drops of almond, coconut, olive, or jojoba oil on your breasts to make it easier to stay in smooth contact with your skin. Remember that some changes in breast tissue condition, appearance, and shape are natural, especially if you are still menstruating. If you are, do your BSE after your period ends and any tenderness or fullness subsides. If you're pregnant, coordinate with your doctor to achieve a new baseline for healthy breasts.

What's normal for you during any stage of your life *is* normal, and you should never have to wonder about variations from the norm in isolation. Share your findings regularly with your doctor, who can help you put them in perspective, based on the many women that he or she examines.

5-Minute Breast Massage

1. Find a private spot at home or elsewhere, and remove your bra (if you're wearing one).
2. With open palms, rub your breasts in a circular motion, in the same direction.
3. Now rotate the breasts in opposite directions.
4. Repeat for up to five minutes.

Consider the breast massage as an antidote to wearing a restrictive bra or sitting for hours at a desk. Manipulating your breasts will jump-start your blood and lymphatic circulation, helping your body do its job of removing toxins. Better yet, create a new habit. Every time you sit on the toilet to pee, put your hands on your breasts and rotate as indicated above.

Yes, Ma'am—Thermogram!

You may be wondering why I waited until now to discuss thermography, an excellent clinical practice for monitoring breast health, in detail. There's a place for everything, and testing should be put in its place. Rather than billing any test as a magical pill for cancer—as the mammogram industry seems to promote *its* service—I want you to think of preventive and diagnostic testing as part of your overall breast health regimen. It's an important part, certainly. But it should complement, not dominate, your personal routine. **Your involvement in your breast health is the best early-warning system for breast cancer that there is.**

Incorporate getting a breast thermogram into your maintenance plan for the right reasons—as a safe way of tracking breast health and heading off cancer development before it takes over. Don't confuse thermogram testing with cancer diagnostics! **Thermograms do not diagnose breast cancer.** For that matter, neither do mammograms, MRIs, or ultrasounds. A diagnosis can only be made by looking under a microscope and seeing cancer cells, or by using a blood test like ONCOblot or RGCC (Research Genetic Cancer Centre). I do not recommend biopsies of single lumps, which would spread the cancer. Single lumps should be excised completely if the thermogram and ultrasound show a high probability of cancer.

Thermograms are a test of physiology, not anatomy like the others. Thermographic imaging was first developed by the U.S. military and was commercially used in industry. It was first employed in breast screening about four decades ago. The FDA approved it for adjunct breast screening in 1982 as a means of helping to detect breast disease. It works by generating real-time footage of lymphatic congestion and temperature patterns in the breasts, using a digital thermal-imaging camera. These cameras capture the infrared light coming from your body as heat, and so are valuable in detecting inflammation and lymphatic congestion that appears as distinct from normal body heat.

Getting a thermogram is not painful or dangerous. Nothing touches or compresses your breasts, and your body is not subjected to harmful x-ray radiation. You might be asked to place your hands in cold water, in order to decrease the base temperature of the breasts, but there will be no smashing or irradiating of tissue.

A breast thermogram is actually a set of seven to nine pictures of your breasts, taken by a thermographer. When you look at a thermogram, you'll see a body outline in colors that correspond to different temperatures in tissue, overlaying gray images of blood vessels in the breast. It looks pretty cool. A certified thermologist reads the results for abnormalities in heat. Simply put, "hot spots" of varying intensity indicate that conditions for breast cancer are developing or could develop.

When you get a thermogram, the reading doctor may use a rating system, which typically runs from *no discernable thermal abnormalities* (TH1) to *thermal abnormalities that indicate very significant risk for breast cancer* (TH5), which puts your results into clinical perspective. Some reading doctors don't use this system. If the thermogram raises concern, then I would recommend, as a next step, an ultrasound.

You do not legally need a prescription to get an ultrasound. However, most ultrasonographers will want one. So find an alternative-care doctor who is willing to recommend an ultrasound for you. The same naturopath, homeopath, or enlightened physician can also prescribe nutritional supplements and lifestyle changes to help you rebalance your system and halt or prevent cancer activity. Now *that's* prevention!

We have already discussed the accuracy (sensitivity and specificity) of thermograms versus mammograms, in Chapter 2. Comparing the two tests, one physiological and one anatomical, is somewhat like comparing apples and oranges. For the purpose that thermograms serve—to identify body conditions that *could* become cancerous—the test comes out far ahead of mammograms in terms of early detection. Once a potential problem is identified, the information gathered by thermography pairs effectively with other anatomical tests, such as ultrasounds and MRIs, neither of which employ radiation.

Thermograms have a distinct advantage over mammograms for younger women and others who have dense breast tissue, which mammograms are notoriously poor at screening. Additionally, **thermograms are the only tests that show pain, inflammation, lymphatic congestion, and the effects of radiation in the breasts.** Inflammation and lymphatic congestion are precursors of cancers and so thermograms are extremely relevant to detecting cancer when it is first developing—something that mammograms simply cannot do.

So, why isn't breast thermography testing used routinely by physicians of all stripes? The infrastructure of trained thermography staff and equipped imaging centers is far less developed than that of mammography; that's why thermogram service can be a challenge to access. I'm not aware of a single source for locating thermographers by region, so to find one, Google "thermography" and your nearest city. For more background on thermograms, please visit my Web site.

How much will it cost? The fee averages between $150–250, not all that much more than the typical mammogram price tag of $100—but thanks to the powers that be, mammograms are fully covered by most insurance plans, and thermograms are not. You pay for mammograms—oh, yes, you do: in your premium—but you don't see the charge. Unless you pay for your thermogram out of pocket, you will probably have to wade through your insurance company's red tape to get a portion of your out-of-network expense reimbursed. A better question than what a thermogram will cost might be what a healthy, long life with two intact breasts is worth. Like I said earlier: easy choice.

Integrated Care

If you want to stay alive and healthy, turning your back on conventional medicine isn't a bad gamble. Researchers at Johns Hopkins Medicine are calling for government health officials to list medical error as the third most common cause of death in America, according to a 2016 report in *The BJM*, a respected British medical journal. This might be an ideal time to embrace complementary and alternative health care!

I have warned you against established medical protocols. I, too, am an MD. I pursued a medical degree to lend additional perspective to what I'd learned as an osteopath (DO) and a naturopathic medical doctor (ND). Having come down the road of integrative medicine myself, I can encourage you to take advantage of health care that comes from different types of providers—those versed in naturopathy, homeopathy, Chinese medicine, conventional Western medicine, or alternative-minded MDs, DOs, and NDs. Take what works for you, and leave the rest. The keys here are to be *healthful* and *safe*. You will have to be the judge of that. So, again, educate yourself, advocate for yourself, and don't stop looking for what works until you find it. Resources for locating alternative-minded DOs or MDs are: www.acam.org or www.worldhealth.net.

Today's atmosphere regarding complementary medicine in America is both accepting and skeptical, depending on which air you're breathing at the moment. The science is solid in some areas—such as regarding the benefits of vitamins, nutraceuticals, and acupuncture—and sparse or nonexistent in others. That's because the pharmaceutical companies drive most of the research. Remember, if they can't make money off a line of inquiry, they steer clear of it.

This is the problem with gaining wider acceptance for many natural treatments: because a particular herb or another natural compound cannot be patented, Big Pharma won't back the research into their potential efficacy . . . unless those elements can be synthesized in a lab and then marketed as proprietary drugs.

More and more women and men, however, are turning to alternative therapies. While one voice might not be heard, eventually consumer demand does break through the medical stalemate, as we have seen. Look at the popularity of taking vitamin C to thwart viruses and cancer, curcumin and SAM-e for inflammation and depression, niacin (vitamin B3) and garlic for blood pressure—and the list goes on and on. There are tens of thousands of published papers on the benefits of vitamins, nutraceuticals, and herbs to prevent or cure disease. However, don't expect your regular doctor to know this, because they were not taught about nutrition or herbals in school—only the use of petroleum-based drugs. Do you want the real story? Take a look at the documentary *That Vitamin Movie.*

The greater number of people taking advantage of bodywork, such as massage, acupuncture, and chiropractic, is another indication of interest in more natural therapies. Those practices were pooh-poohed for ages by the medical establishment—until the right researchers found proof of their health benefits.

What I've found in my practice of integrative medicine is that many of the protocols that do the least physical damage—and make the establishment the least profit—are ideal for treating patients with breast cancer. Because the odds of developing this disease are significant, you will want to know more about this kinder, gentler way of leading women back to health. I invite you to learn from my experiences in healing patients over the years.

Are you ready? Then turn the page.

11 Suspicion, Detection, and Perspective

... If Breast Cancer Affects You (or Someone You Love)

Even if you never have illness associated with your breasts, given the incidence rates, an acquaintance or loved one of yours likely will. You can apply the news in this section to your own life or share it, if the right moment arises. You can't force advice on people, especially when they are already swimming in it.

The moment folks learn that you might be sick, they come out of the woodwork with solutions. We all have that urge to help—because we care, certainly, but also because it makes us feel less vulnerable. An emotional response to cancer, however, won't help, at this point. Knowledge will. You have picked up this book because you are ready to listen and learn, and that gives you power.

If you suspect or are diagnosed with breast cancer, being open to new ideas will be a big plus. Openness to information is not the same as grasping at straws. It is a way to wade through conflicting advice—good and bad, reasonable and questionable—on the subject of breast cancer. Think *options*, because you are going to need them, from diagnosis to treatment. Every case is individual. But the conventional health care community doesn't always see it that way. Doctors who are closed to what works for different women have just a few straws to grasp at, anyhow.

To make up for a dearth of diagnosis and treatment options, the medical establishment pushes haste. Hurry to get another mammogram; hurry to get a biopsy. *Quick! Start chemotherapy and radiation . . .* before you have time to research and learn that there are many other options. Speed appeals to patients who are in a panic. On the surface, it makes sense to get timely help. But if that "help" is harmful to your condition (which may not be cancer), and if that urgent schedule does not correlate with the pace of actual cancer growth, then that advice does not make sense—nor will it improve your chances of getting well.

Rush to biopsy? Rush to chemo, radiation, or surgery? *No, ma'am.* Never mind what your initial reflex is, your first move should be to take a step back. **Do not rush into a critical medical decision.** Instead, arm yourself with knowledge, so you can choose your course of healing wisely. It is shameful that medical professionals will not encourage this, although it is natural on their parts to try to maintain their authority.

Think of the pressure to act, the limited solutions that are offered, and your vast lack of wisdom on the topic of breast cancer as a towering wall between you and healing. If you stand right next to the wall—which is where doctors will push you—you can't see over it. All kinds of solutions might be waiting for you right there, on the other side. But, if you are overwhelmed by pressure and with fear and panic, you go where those things lead you: off on the wrong tangent and into a downward spiral. How can you move forward until you know where to put your feet? By taking a step back to gather your wits and all the information you can find on your condition, you'll be able to see over the wall!

Such perspective is a real gain. So, press PAUSE. Pausing is not a lack of progress, as doctors would have you think, but a critical element of a proper decision.

If you receive a suspicious test result, or one that indicates breast cancer as highly likely, certainly, take action. Go to work. Go to work on becoming the most informed person on Planet Earth about your condition. It's *yours.* It's not one size fits all, it's not what your friends and family say it is; it is in your body, so *you* apply everything you can possibly learn about it to your circumstances. Then you can make decisions. Then you can accept and try out solutions. You can't control your diagnosis, but you can control your approach to healing.

Now is the time to be firm about who's in charge. You may be deluged with helpful (and nonhelpful) hints and offers of solace from the people in your life. Accept their care—their hearts are in the right place—but you do not have to accept their intervention. We are conditioned toward instant gratification in this culture and often forget that we do not have to answer every question or act on every piece of advice right away. When you are faced with well-meaning inquiries and unsolicited advice from people, thank them and say you'll have to think about it, and you'll get back to them about what you decide. Setting boundaries now will keep you in charge and guide you through what's to come.

If you choose to go the alternative route, expect severe pressure from family and friends. You will need to be very clear with them from the get-go: *If you cannot support me, then do not engage me. If you are going to resist me, please get out of my life for this period of time.* Do not get hung up on being nice. Right now, boundaries are critical, both to your mental state and your freedom to choose how to heal *your* body.

Here is one way to lay out the ground rules. When doctors, friends, or relatives demand that you do what they want you to do—right now—tell them: "This is my game. I am the coach, and I am the manager. If you want to play on my team, you get to come into the game if and when I decide that's best for me. Until then, you are on the bench. My life, my body, my team. Are you with me?"

Good to know . . .

Chemotherapy, drugs administered intravenously or orally, usually including chemical compounds developed to kill rapidly dividing cells.
Radiation therapy, targeted x-ray radiation exposure intended to kill cells in cancerous masses.
Mastectomy, surgical removal of part or all of the breast.

Why Biopsies (and Chemo and Radiation) Suck

If you find a lump in your breast during a self-exam, stop looking for what could be wrong, and start seeking perspective. There are many reasons to take it slow and be positive. Think back to when things were "normal." What has changed?

Let's begin with your first inkling that something is amiss with your breasts. Your inner knower senses a shift in your body. Is that cancer? No. You can't say yet that it is. Pain, lumps, fluid accumulation, changes in appearance—these may accompany malignancy, but they may also be signs of noncancerous cysts, adenomas, or calcifications, which are various types of tissue states. How will you find out?

Let's say you talk to your regular doctor, who checks the lump and immediately wants to order a mammogram x-ray, to determine whether it is a fluid-filled cyst or a hard-mass tumor. You request an ultrasound, to avoid the radiation, but are told that you must have a mammogram first, and then an ultrasound to augment its findings.

Why?

Ultrasounds have a good track record in testing to distinguish cysts from tumors. To my knowledge, there is no insurance regulation or law in any state requiring a mammogram before ultrasound; it's just what the medical system does. Doctors work under "standard of care" protocols, or, supposedly, what's best to try first, second, third, and so on. The sellers of mammography machines have seen to it that mammograms are the first item on that list for breast problems, even though scientific data clearly indicates that it is an inferior test and, indeed, *causes* cancer. So the doctors who echo that "standard of care" when you ask for an ultrasound instead of a mammogram first are being good lemmings and not thinking for themselves. So ask yourself the question, Why should you undergo cancer-causing radiation exposure if your condition is benign? Could it be that promoting cancer will perpetuate your need for medical care?

If you cannot get cooperation in scheduling your ultrasound without a mammogram, then you may have to work around that problem. Go ahead and cooperate: schedule both tests, say, on the same day or a day apart. When the mammogram appointment comes up, just call and reschedule it. Then, go get the ultrasound and, later, cancel the mammogram, saying you decided not to go that route. If the system is unhappy, then so be it. Also, you do not legally need a prescription to get an ultrasound. If your doctor doesn't request one, you can request one, although you may have to pay for it yourself.

Now, suppose you make it over that hurdle and a mass *is* detected. Go back to putting things in perspective. While the possibility of serious illness exists, it has not been confirmed or denied. Take charge of what you can, and adjust your diet and lifestyle as if you do have cancer, but remind yourself that—at the moment, as far as you know—you are healthy and unencumbered. Even though breast cancer numbers are significant, nine out of ten breast lumps are *not* cancerous. You might have one of these instead:

- **Fibrous cyst,** a persistent condition among 60 percent of all women, characterized by harmless fibrous lumps
- **Fluid-filled cyst,** sacs of fluid in breast tissue that are often tender or painful, common to about 30 percent of women age 35 to 50
- **Fibroadenoma,** a benign tumor of smooth, hard, rubbery consistency that moves within the breast tissue (as opposed to malignant tumors that are rough and rooted within tissue)
- **Calcification,** a calcium deposit that usually appears in groups, which may arise from clogged milk ducts or arteries, injury, or inflammation due to infection

What is it? Any solid mass should be identified. Your doctor will probably push you to get a confirmation mammogram and then a biopsy. Politely say, "No, ma'am!" and request an MRI first. This test will reveal more about the lump's size, consistency, and location, but won't definitively diagnose malignancy. If the thermogram, ultrasound, and MRI are highly suspicious, I would recommend removing the lump without a biopsy.

In any case, refuse a needle biopsy if you have a solitary lump. A breast mass of 1 cm has about 1 billion cells in it. If this mass is cancerous, then driving a high-speed metal projectile (biopsy needle) through the lump of cancer cells, cutting across veins and lymph vessels, blowing cancer cells off, and then drawing the needle back through the normal tissue is not a good idea. You now have loose cancer cells and vessels that have been cut, allowing these cells to spread within your body instantly. There has never been a double-blind study showing that biopsies decrease death rates from cancer! Just take out the lump. If your doctor will not agree to this, then change doctors!

Conventional tests may also spread a type of breast cancer that is not harmful or aggressive as long as it stays where it is. Ductal carcinoma *in situ,* or DCIS, inhabits the milk ducts. This condition accounts for 75 percent of all diagnosed breast cancers, and it does not need to be eliminated, just prevented from migrating. The compression of mammogram plates and invasion of biopsy needles, however, can cause DCIS cells to move from the ducts to tissue served by the lymphatic system—and from there, it travels where it will. So, while biopsies and mammograms can give you hard answers, they can also create a life-threatening situation where one did not previously exist.

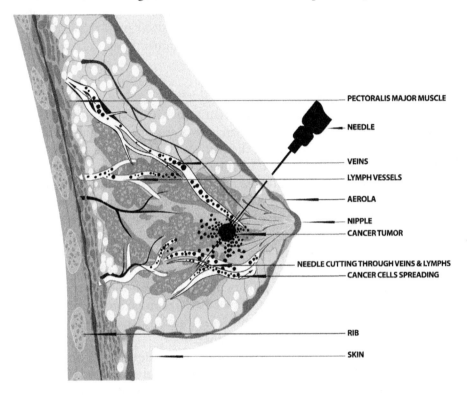

Another diagnostic option is to remove the full lump for analysis, a surgical procedure called a lumpectomy, for which patients are anesthetized. This is the only way to diagnose breast cancer for sure without harming the rest of your body. However, if the lab does find cancer, standard protocol is to immediately remove the breast, theoretically removing the cancer, while you are still under anesthesia. The primary reason for that is, having done a biopsy first, they *know* they have already spread the cancer locally. If you have not had a biopsy and are electing to do a lumpectomy, then **DO NOT** sign the papers that would allow them to do a mastectomy. Press PAUSE. You can decide this later after additional testing. And who knows whether cancer cells have spread elsewhere in numbers too small to detect?

Rather than opt for lumpectomies—and, if cancer is found, the preemptive loss of a breast—I personally favor early-intervention treatment over disturbing the mass. Leaving the lump there and monitoring it will tell you whether your therapies are working. Surgery should be a last resort. Suppose you acquiesce to chemotherapy and radiation. Without the visible evidence of a tumor shrinking or growing, how will you know whether your treatment is effective?

The same logic holds true if you choose to adopt homeopathic or other complementary therapies. While you pursue them, your physician can use information gathered from thermograms and blood tests to assess the state of your health and the presence of cancer. Meanwhile, you can address any breast inflammation by applying a castor oil or flaxseed oil pack daily. The plant compounds in these oils naturally reduce inflammation and act to suppress cancer growth.

Alternatives *Are* Better

Suppose you have started down the conventional road after a positive diagnosis. Your doctor will lay out a treatment plan in response to your symptoms instead of what caused your condition in the first place. The rush to chemotherapy and radiation therapy is based on killing cancer cells, not on fixing things. Furthermore, the side effects of those protocols **severely damage the immune system**, your body's natural means of fighting off disease. You should be allowed to pursue healing through methods that work with your body, not against it.

The Achilles heel of chemotherapy and radiation is that they damage the immune system. Let me help you understand, chemo and/or radiation will never kill 100 percent of the cancer cells. At the end of the day, your immune system has to be functioning to pick up the slack, or you will not survive. Why does the lab always check your white blood cell count before your next chemo or radiation treatment? To see if this "cure" has so damaged your immune system that they can't give you the next dose.

But herbal, homeopathic, and metabolic treatments and lifestyle adjustments take time—probably much longer than the standard six-to seven-week blasts of chemicals or radiation that your regular doctor offers. If the price of swift intervention is the loss of immune function, that's a raw deal. We'll talk more about that in a moment. Consider what your time frame really is.

First of all, how was your cancer identified? By evidence in a mammogram? As we have seen, masses of 0.5 to 1 cm that are detectable by mammography take eight to ten years to reach that size. When patients call me with a newly diagnosed cancer, the first thing I tell them is that they do not have to make a decision today, this week, or this month. Study and learn about your specific condition. Investigate all the possibilities. Seek the counsel of someone who loves you and is open to alternatives. Seek divine guidance; then make your decision.

Retaining your body's natural ability to destroy cancer cells **and to recover afterwards** is crucial, no matter what treatment you choose. Chemo and radiation therapies do not eliminate cancer in your body; they kill a portion of the billions of cancer cells present, leaving the rest to continue dividing and growing. Radiation, itself, *causes* further cancer. That is where immune defense comes in.

Natural killer cells, a type of white blood lymphocytes, are a part of your immune system designed to allow you to overcome cancer. Thanks to our tainted environment and lifestyles, we all get cancer every day; a robust immune system simply denies it the opportunity to take hold. If it does and your treatment suppresses lymphocyte production and other immune functions, your body will not be able to fend off the cancer cells that chemo and radiation miss.

Not only that, focusing solely on killing cancer cells discounts what encouraged them to form in the first place. Here is where moving into complementary or alternative care is the superior route. You will never hear conventional doctors ask "what caused" your cancer. Therefore, they only treat the result, not the cause. Even if they do help you win the battle, that doesn't mean you have won the war. If the cause remains, your cancer can return. The biggest lie is, "We got it all."

Say *Adieu,* Not *Au Revoir,* to Cancer

There are many books that will help you understand in more detail how breast cancer develops and how conventional medical treatments affect the body. Other sources, including *The Secret of Health: Breast Wisdom*, which I coauthored, describe the science behind complementary and alternative health modalities. This knowledge, coupled with statistics on costs and survival rates, will tell you which options are viable for you. My aim in this book is to help you take the right steps back to breast health. This means identifying the root cause of cancer, and reversing or eliminating it. That is how you will say *farewell* to cancer, not *see you next time*.

Despite all that I have shared with you in these chapters, when you are recovering from cancer is no time to DIY. To assess where you're at, I recommend Jenny Hrbacek's book: *Cancer Free! Are You Sure?* For professional help, seek the guidance of a naturopathic doctor (ND or NMD) who is trained in nutrition and homeopathy, or an integrative oncologist, like myself, who pairs a specialty in cancer treatment with natural medicine. These professionals can suggest nutritional and herbal supplements that will be effective for your specific condition. See the Appendix for a list of what an alternative care physician should be able to provide. Interventions may include:

- **Hormone therapy,** using natural estriol to occupy estrogen receptor sites that promote cancer growth instead of Tamoxifen
- **Carbon dioxide therapy,** which reduces blood acidity and optimizes oxygen delivery

- **Ozone therapy,** which lowers viral, fungal and bacterial loads
- **Dietary modifications,** to help "starve" cancer cells and bolster the immune system
- **Massage therapy,** to relieve pain and stimulate lymphatic circulation
- **Mental health therapy,** in individual or group discussion sessions, to overcome emotional stress

There are women for whom this news may seem to come too late. If you've always gone to regular medical doctors and have taken their advice for treating cancer, coping with the recovery period after chemo and radiation therapies will be tough. You're basically back to square one—sick and at the mercy of limiting medical advice. Don't let yourself be boxed in by your first treatment choice. Now is the time to start over anyway, so go ahead and take advantage of what we've discussed so far. You don't have to do it all at once.

To help you make the leap from chemo and radiation to more positive healing, here are two easy first steps. First, to counteract the effects of the drugs and radiation on your immune system, take maximum recommended doses of high-quality antioxidant supplements, such as: vitamins A, C, and E; alpha lipoic acid (ALA); pycnogenol, which is derived from pine tree bark; and green tea extract. You can purchase all of these in capsule form from a vitamin shop.

Second, forget what your doctor has told you about diet and weight at this time. Routine counsel is to eat whatever you like to keep up your strength. True, you don't want to drop too much weight when you have cancer, but do eat the right foods to maintain it. My best recommendation is to cut out the sugar and carbs—cancer cells love the glucose that they provide—and concentrate on eating healthy fats, which carry twice the calories of sugar and carbs per gram. Avocados, oily fish, and any seed or nut oils are great sources, or just munch on walnuts, sunflower seeds, or pumpkin seeds. This advice is good for all recovering cancer patients, but can particularly help those who have been set back by chemical or radiation damage.

In order to leave cancer behind and restore your well-being, take advantage of all of your personal resources and the healthy options available to you. If you haven't yet made the move to organic foods, doing so now will be a concrete step in the right direction that will also offset any trouble you might be having with your appetite. Choose high-quality protein sources, like wild-caught fish and lean, hormone- and GMO-free meat. Even if food doesn't appeal to you or you can't eat much, at least you will know that what you are getting is good for you. You can add an unflavored protein powder, or one sweetened with stevia or xylitol, to whatever you eat, for extra support to your immune system. Be sure to get some sunshine, fresh air, and exercise as often as possible, too.

One of your best healthy resources is your network of like-minded friends and family. Emotional and practical support significantly raises cancer survival rates. Get together with friends to laugh and cry. Spend time with your pets. Encourage your partner to find support, too, so you won't be plagued by guilt over what he or she has to endure. You need all your energy to repair the damage wrought by cancer and medical treatments. The best thing you can do for yourself at this time is to ask for and accept help—from companionship to housecleaning and relief from other daily obligations. That's what your loved ones are for. But remember, if they can't support what you have chosen, get them out of your life temporarily.

There is one more major recommendation that I have to offer, which will apply before, during, and after you have any issues with the health of your breasts. We've discussed how important your thoughts and intentions are to achieving and maintaining health. This moral and spiritual ground becomes even more critical if you are ill, recovering, or attempting to prevent a return of breast cancer. Let's take a final look at the Law of Attraction that so influences your health, next.

12 Live Your Life in Love

Parting Words

Sometimes we don't try a new thing—or know if that thing will positively influence us—until we experience adversity. Back when I was still focusing on family practice, I had a vague awareness of, and interest in, alternative care. But it wasn't until my cancer patients came to me asking, "What about this nutritional or nutraceutical? What about vitamins?" that I began to realize my limitations. There were many natural things out there that would bring about health and wellness without using drugs. It was then that I began to pursue a naturopathic degree and look into new ways of healing the body that had not been covered in medical school.

Even so, I did not fully apply what I learned to my own life until tragedy struck. In 2002 I was diagnosed with amyotrophic lateral sclerosis (ALS), or Lou Gehrig's disease. My symptoms had begun as occasional muscle tremors and progressed to near-constant contractions beneath my skin that were clearly visible. I was overcome with fatigue, and I became so weak that I could barely speak or walk from here to there.

An orthopedic surgeon diagnosed my condition, and a second opinion confirmed it: I had ALS, a progressive illness of the motor nerves that carries a prognosis of death. Eighty percent of people with ALS die within five years; about one in ten makes it beyond ten years.

I knew from my experience in the conventional medical world that there was no hope for me there. And, in my complementary practice, I had treated ALS patients in the past. But neither herbal, nutritional, nor homeopathic remedies had helped; my recommendations for energy work and acupuncture did not affect the disease progression. Any door to my options appeared to be closed.

A few months later—during which I'd begun preparing for my death—I met Dr. Alex Loyd, a naturopath and psychologist who held some very interesting ideas about treating the cause of illness. Based on the desire to help his wife overcome debilitating depression, as I have mentioned, he developed a system that applies quantum physics to remove the effects of stress on the body at the cellular level. He calls this method The Healing Codes, and it can be directed to whichever part of the body most needs it.

The premise is that the effects of physical and mental stress can form any number of combinations on cellular memory that may stress our immune system, making it unable to respond to emerging disease. Address those instigators, and you can heal illness.

Both the scientific and practical logic of this theory appealed to me. I cast off my preparations for the end and began learning and applying The Health Codes technique. This involves saying a prayer for healing and using certain hand positions to direct your physical energy through the body, in specific sequences at specific portals.

In the space of six weeks, my muscle twitches and other symptoms began to wane. In eight weeks, they were gone, and I felt that the degeneration in my body had ceased and that I had begun to recover.

Proof Positive

I did recover my health to enjoy a happy, active existence. It has been fourteen years since my ALS symptoms began, and thirteen since they departed. I sometimes feel an involuntary muscular twitch or two, which serves to renew my resolve to avoid the kind of emotional stress that prompted my sickness. As I mentioned before, people tend to dwell on the downside of life. This isn't just an unpleasant habit; it has very real consequences! My primary guideline, then and now, is to turn away from the negative aspects in myself, other people, and daily events, and to live from the heart. It's not a state of denial, but one of conscious acceptance—of the positive things in life.

I share this story with you not to suggest that you do exactly as I did if you are taken ill, but to encourage you to be open to the concepts behind my actions. Yes, The Healing Codes unlocked my system and allowed me to get well. Had I not been open to new ideas, however, I would never have availed myself of that chance. I say *open* in the sense of being willing to hear Dr. Loyd out and give his process a try, and perhaps more importantly, being willing to believe that I could get better.

I needed both of those motivations, because you cannot fool the cells of your body. Just as dramatized images that you've seen are embedded in your cellular memory as truth, so are your negative feelings. Any skepticism that I harbored over my ability to survive would have surfaced as physical stress, blocking my application of The Healing Codes and further wearing down my immune system. This episode showed me that my outlook on life and my degree of integrity have everything to do with ongoing health. It wasn't enough to just get well. I had to *be* well. So, apart from my successful recovery, I would have to work at retaining that positive emotional state . . . for the rest of my life.

It is this tool with which I wish to leave you: the power to allow your body to function as it was so ingeniously designed. I believe **disease can**

arise when the effects of mental and physical stress block the efforts of the immune system to restore balance and well-being to the body. If we avoid the sources of this stress, or at least prevent wrong beliefs and other negative influences from piling up within our cellular memory, we can stay healthy.

Think of this captured stress like the chemical toxins that invade your system. Your liver can handle a certain volume of contaminants per day, such as low levels of chlorine or isolated incidences of bacterial poisoning. But when your toxic load gets too high—say, from drinking polluted water day after day—your body can't slough off all the residue. This mirrors the effect of long-term stress on the cells of the body.

I have already told you how to avoid concrete external forms of stress, from bad water to microwaves to mammogram x-rays. And we've discussed working with the Law of Attraction in an effort to draw positive energy into your life and repel negative things, like illness. Remember that forgiveness is a catalyst to this undertaking: in letting go of old friction, you make space for the good stuff. I also confessed that this is a difficult thing to do, and a task that may never be "done."

It helps if you forgive yourself first. Untangle your emotional strings to whatever regrets most haunt you—things you've done, things didn't do, or things you wished you'd done. Within these memories are feelings of guilt, anger, and embarrassment, some of which you've been holding onto for years. To what end? Whether you did or did not make amends, or whether you plan to, does not change the past. It's over.

Make your final step toward breast health one of contemplation. Take some time to sit down and unearth the things that you most blame yourself for, and find a way to release them. Accept that you learned something from the situation, so you can now seek peace. Or, if feelings of unworthiness get in the way, dissociate yourself from the equation. Forgive that "other" person in you; this might help you see yourself more clearly and, ultimately, be able to forgive others.

I want you to do this periodically, to clear your emotional channels and ignite your spiritual energy. Doing so gives you the power to move purposefully where your heart leads you.

To stay well, my best advice is to live well. Live fully. Have faith. Remember that it is in giving that you receive, and that whatever you sow, you reap. So give joyfully and sow plentifully. Live in hope. Even greater "medicine" than faith and hope, though, is love. **Resolve to live your life in love.** From that will flow good health—to your breasts, to your mind, and to your body.

About the Author

Ben Johnson, MD, DO, NMD, is an integrative oncologist who is recognized worldwide as a leader in complementary medicine. A renowned speaker on natural healing, he was featured in the 2006 documentary and best-selling book, *The Secret*. Born in North Georgia, he now lives and works in San Diego, California.

Dr. Ben combines expertise gained as a medical doctor, osteopath, and naturopathic medical doctor with alternative approaches to healing cancer on a concierge basis, in which he cares for patients in the comfort of their homes. He focused in general practice for many years, and served as senior flight surgeon for the U.S. Army Reserve and as senior aviation medical examiner (AME) for the Federal Aviation Administration. Dr. Ben currently serves as the Minister of Health for the Southern Cherokee Nation RFP. In addition to his medical degrees, he holds a B.S. in biology and M.S. in psychology.

To promote the cause of early cancer detection, Dr. Ben founded the International Cancer Foundation and co-founded Thermography Unlimited. He is the author of *Healing Waters* and coauthor of *The Healing Code* and *The Secret of Health: Breast Wisdom*. Readers can find a wealth of educational materials on breast health, breast cancer, and healthy living by visiting Dr. Ben's Web site at www.drbenmd.com.

Resources

Thank you for your interest in this work. In appreciation, Dr. Ben would like to offer you a free video series on important health issues. To receive this, please visit www.drbenmd.com/offer.

To continue to be updated on important health information, visit www.drbenmd.com.

Here is a list of additional valuable resources:

www.universalmedicalimaging.com
www.truthaboutcancer.com
www.mercola.com
www.healthrangerreport.com
www.cancerdecisions.com
www.greenmedinfo.com
www.bestanswerforcancer.org

Appendix

These are some of the treatment options that your alternative physician should probably have in their toolbox:

2-DG (2-Deoxy-D-glucose). A hexokinase II (HK2) inhibitor that can cause cell death by competing with glucose in the energy the cycle.

3BP (3-Bromopyruvate). Another HK2 inhibitor, which kills cancer cells without damaging normal cells and is then broken down and leaves the body without any remaining toxicity.

5-Azacytidine. Macrophage activating factor (MAF). Can be used to stimulate the immune system back into action.

Cesium Chloride. Alkalinizes the blood and is toxic to cancer cells.

DMSO. Helps to get therapeutics into cancer cells and is itself an anti-cancer agent.

EDTA. Used to remove the heavy metals that decrease immune response, which are present in everybody's system.

Estriol. Can be used to occupy estrogen receptor sites instead of Tamoxifen.

Fatty Acid Synthase Inhibitor. Prevents cancer cells from using fatty acids as fuel.

Germanium Sesquioxide. A cancer-cell killer.

IPT/LDC. Insulin Pontentiated Therapy with low-dose chemo. Small doses of IV insulin open up cancer cells and close normal cells, so that a tiny dose of chemo can be driven into cancer cells without damaging white blood cells, the liver, the heart, etc.

Lonidamine. Increases lactic acid in cancer cells, causing cell death there but not damaging white blood cells or normal cells.

Methylglyoxal. Helps degrade the energy production cycle of cancer cells.

Naltrexone. Drug that helps recovering alcoholics; has been found useful in cancer in small doses.

Ozone. Lowers viral, bacterial, fungal, and cancer loads in the body.

Progesterone. Slows cancer-cell replication rate.

Sodium Bicarbonate. Alkalinizes the blood so that it can carry more oxygen.

Vitamin C. Has been known to treat cancer successfully.

About Radical Rethink

Radical Rethink is a series of books written to create awareness and education on topics that have not been addressed accurately by conventional medicine. The standard of care is limited to surgery, drugs, and radiation, when most conditions are preventable and treatable with herbs, nutritionals, homeopathics, and energy medicine.

Dr. Ben's follow up book to *No Ma'am-ogram!* will be on Alzheimer's disease. It will provide very valuable information to treat this insidious disease naturally, without the prescription drugs that cause additional damage to the body and don't even come close to treating the condition. Through extensive research, Dr. Ben has learned that Alzheimer's is actually reversible.

Stay tuned for other upcoming books that will entice you to radically rethink everything you've ever learned!

Dr. Ben will be including real stories from patients who have suffered and experienced the dark side of the medical establishment and he would love to hear from you. Please send your stories to info@drbenmd.com.

"For lack of knowledge, my people perish"
~ Hosea 4:6

SELECT BIBLIOGRAPHY

Allen, Marshall and Olga Pierce. "Medical Errors are No. 3 Cause of U.S. Deaths, Researchers Say. National Public Radio Online, published May 3, 2016. http://www.npr.org/sections/health-shots/2016/05/03/476636183/death-certificates-undercount-toll-of-medical-errors.

Diakides, Nicholas A. and Joseph D. Bronzino, eds. *Medical Infrared Imaging*. Boca Raton, FL: Taylor & Francis, 2008.

Gannon, Megan. "Antibacterial Soap Ingredient May Cause Cancer in Mice." Live Science, published November 19, 2014. http://www.livescience.com/48822-triclosan-exposure-caused-liver-cancer-mice.html.

Gøtzsche, Peter. *Mammography Screening: Truth, Lies and Controversy.* London: Radcliffe, 2012.

Harding, Charles, et al. "Breast Cancer Screening, Incidence, and Mortality Across US Counties." *JAMA Intern Med.* 2015; 175(9): 1483-1489.

Horner, MD, FACS, Christine. *Waking the Warrior Goddess: Dr. Christine Horner's Program to Protect Against & Fight Breast Cancer.* Laguna Beach, CA: Basic Health, 2007.

Johnson, MD, DO, NMD, Ben. *Healing Waters: The Powerful Health Benefits of Ionized H20.* Garden City Park, NY: Square One, 2011.

Johnson, MD, DO, NMD, Ben and Kathleen Barnes. *The Secret of Health: Breast Wisdom.* Garden City, NY: Morgan James, 2008.

Malkan, Stacy. "Johnson & Johnson Is Just the Tip of the Toxic Iceberg." Time Online, published March 2, 2016. http://time.com/4239561/johnson-and-johnson-toxic-ingredients.

Singer, Sydney Ross and Soma Grismaijer. *Dressed to Kill: The Link Between Breast Cancer and Bras.* Pahoa, HI: ISCD Press, 2006.

Womenshealth.gov. "Mammograms Fact Sheet." Last modified June 21, 2013. http://womenshealth.gov/publications/our-publications/fact-sheet/mammograms.html.